Angel With Broken Wings

The Story of Basil Rhodes, Jr.

Dorothy Rhodes

with

Deb Johnson

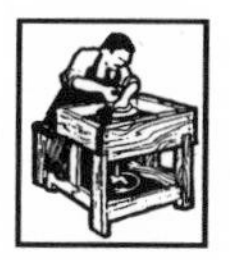

Guild Press of Indiana
Indianapolis IN 46208

Library of Congress Number 95-81759

ISBN: 1-878208-78-0

CONTENTS

PROLOGUE

This is a true story about a brave and courageous young man named Basil W. Rhodes, Jr. Basil was born with a rare bone disease called Osteogenesis Imperfecta which left him severely handicapped. He was a great inspiration to family, friends, and community.

He was also an achiever. Basil was an honor student who received his schooling at home with a homebound teacher, who would go to the school in which Basil was enrolled and get his lesson plans a week at a time.

He won an award in tenth grade for getting the highest score on a standardized government test. With the aid of tutors, he graduated ninth in his Bluffton High School class.

His perseverance through pain and incredible difficulties was well recognized. Basil was the first person in Indiana to receive the Young Heroes' Medal of Honor award for: "Having Shown Outstanding Courage and Valor." The award was presented to Basil on behalf of the officers and airmen of the HQ 122nd Tactical Fighter Wing Indiana Air National Guard on the twenty-eighth day of August, 1991, at the Fort Wayne Indiana Air Base.

Basil was always a joy to be with. He loved playing Nintendo, watching I.U. basketball games, going shopping at the mall and listening to his Christian rock music. Basil enjoyed life abundantly; even though his pain was unspeakable, he never complained.

Basil said, "God put me here for a reason. I am who I am and I like it! If we could all accept and like ourselves, then we would be much happier."

As Basil's mother, I'm sure his closeness with God has made him a very happy and special angel in heaven with no more pain and suffering. Certainly he was our angel on earth.

Dorothy Rhodes
December, 1995

INTRODUCTION TO BASIL'S FAMILY

The story of Basil actually started eleven years before his birth. Basil Sr. and I met through the friendship of our dads. Both of our fathers worked in the timber business in Ripley, West Virginia. In 1963, our home burned down; my dad ended up buying a house that Mr. Rhodes had built. Shortly after that, the Rhodes family rented a house just up the hill from us; now we were neighbors. Basil and I met through his brothers, Gary and Arles, who came to our house a lot after school. One day Basil stopped in, and Gary introduced us. Since I was only thirteen and Basil was nineteen, my dad would not allow us to date. "Dorothy," he said, "Basil's a grown man and you're just a kid in diapers."

After we finally got to date when I was sixteen, Basil was drafted and had to serve in Vietnam. I was a junior in high school then; that was also the year my parents divorced.

I had come to know Basil as a caring, kind man. This quality was one of the first things that attracted me to Basil. I soon realized just how caring he was. After the divorce, Basil made certain that I got everything I needed, from a new winter coat to my senior pictures. Even when he was in Vietnam, he had asked his mother to make sure that I had anything I needed. He returned home on July 4, 1967. Because he needed a job, he moved to Bluffton, Indiana, to work at Corning Glass; his brother, Gary, had been working there since he graduated from high school. At that point, we were engaged, but we had not yet set a date to be married. He could only come home once a month when he had a five-day break from work. But we sure kept the phone lines hot! We knew we were meant for each other. Basil was a workaholic, and still is to this day. I am more people-oriented so we balance each other. We finally married September 15, 1968.

After our wedding in West Virginia, we moved up to Bluffton, so Basil could continue working at Corning Glass. He worked there seventeen years, until the company closed down the factory, and during that time, Basil had the opportunity of traveling to China, India, and Mexico to train the employees of the newly-opened factories. As soon as he received notice that the factory would be closing, Basil bought a semi and he was on the road the week after the plant shut down; taught by my brother, Jim, he learned the basics of driving the truck. Basil drove for about a year, and then ended up in another factory, Isolatek International, in Huntington, Indiana, where he still works twelve-hour shifts, three days one week, and four days the next week. Remember when I mentioned that he was a great provider and workaholic? He has always worked every spare moment, needing very little sleep. His extra work involves construction.

I, too, worked at Corning after we were married, for ten years. Basil and I worked the same shift, and a baby-sitter came to stay with Priscilla. After Basil Jr. was born, my mom stayed with the kids while we worked. I worked at Corning until 1978 when Basil built a new house for us in the country. Then I went to work off and on at Meadowvale Care Center, a nursing home in Bluffton, which I enjoyed. I also worked as a teacher's aide at Adams-Wells Co-Op, a school for mentally and physically handicapped children. This was just a couple miles north of our home, so it was convenient for me if I needed to get home quickly for Basil Jr.

In 1971, our family had grown with the birth of our daughter, Priscilla. I had trouble with my pregnancy; at five weeks, I had to take a leave from work, and experienced trouble with bleeding, for which I had to receive shots. The delivery went smoothly, and we had a lovely six-pound eleven-ounce daughter who turned into a pretty, happy girl. She was definitely a daddy's girl; I guess she still is today. When Basil worked nights, he'd often take Priscilla with him during the day. One of her favorite things was to ride the motorcycle with her daddy.

When Priscilla was two, I found out I was pregnant, again. I had to take leave from work, again, and I had to take the same bleeding-control injections, but more frequently, sometimes twice a week. Priscilla was very excited about being a big sister. I told her all the ways she could help when the baby came—bathing, diapers, and feeding. She could hardly wait for the day! Little did I know that because of an unexpected turn of events, these normally simple tasks would be terribly difficult for me as a mother, and nearly impossible for Priscilla as a sister.

THE BIRTH OF BASIL

I can remember my pregnancy with Basil Jr. as if it were yesterday. It seemed as though I spent about as much time at the hospital as I did at home, trying to prevent a hemorrhage which would have made me lose the baby. This nearly happened when I was five months pregnant.

I expressed my concern about all the complications I was having, plus the fact that the baby seldom moved. My doctor replied, "Dorothy, you're worrying over nothing. The baby is normal size, and you should never compare one pregnancy with another. They're all different, but I'm sure you're going to have a healthy baby." To this day I don't know how or why, but I knew there would be a problem with my child at birth.

I will always remember my thoughts and conversation with God. I said, "Oh, Lord, I don't mean to choose, or to seem ungrateful toward this wonderful child you are giving me. But I do feel there is something wrong since the child seldom moves. I know, Lord, you will not put more burden on me than I can handle. So please, Lord, if there is a serious problem, let it be anything but a mental handicap. But if that is how life has to be, Lord, I'll love the child and do the best I can every day we have together. Just look after the both of us every day, Heavenly Father."

As the next four months progressed, everything remained the same. Then on March 4th at 3:00 AM, my labor started with Basil Jr. I got my husband up from a sound sleep; he took Priscilla to a friend's house. By the time he got home I was dressed and ready for the hospital.

After I'd been admitted into the hospital and all the pre-delivery care was given, my doctor came in to examine me. That is when I discovered Basil was breech. During delivery, my contractions suddenly stopped. The doctor sent for medication to start the contractions again. I overheard a nurse nervously whispering, "We have to get the baby out, or it will smother to death!" Upon hearing that, I became terrified. I was so upset that the doctor quite firmly told me, "Young lady, you get hold of yourself. You have to help me here!" As soon as I received the medication, the pains started back up. It was a difficult delivery; he was born with a broken arm and leg. The X-ray showed many broken bones that Basil had during the pregnancy; he had endured the pain of broken bones and of the healing process before he was even born. At birth, Basil weighed six pounds, five ounces, and was sixteen inches long; he had long black hair on his small, perfectly rounded head. It was several hours, though, before they brought him to me. They were taking X-rays and the doctors were examining him. It sounds strange, but I never really became hysterical during those long hours. I had suspected all along that something was wrong with my baby; I knew that whatever it was, I would deal with it and that God would help me. When Basil was finally brought into my room, he was on a pillow because he was so fragile. That's how I carried him for several years.

I feel very fortunate that Dr. Pat Bader was working in the research building connected with Caylor Nickel Clinic during the time of Basil's birth. She was the doctor who diagnosed him as having Osteogenesis Imperfecta. Looking into his eyes revealed to her the devastating disease with which he was born. The whites of Basil's eyes were blue; this is known as blue sclera and is a characteristic of this disease. Osteogenesis Imperfecta, or OI, is a genetic disorder where the collagen in the bones does not form. This leaves the victim's bones hard and brittle, not allowing for normal bone growth. A child with OI could remain the physical size of a year-old baby all of his or her life.

OI AND RELATED PROBLEMS

Various syndromes are associated with Osteogenesis Imperfecta. Common characteristics include short stature, blue sclera, and poorly formed dentin; however, it is the susceptibility to fractures that causes most of the clinical problems for the patient. The severe form of OI is manifest at birth, as in Basil's case. A less severe form may not show up until later years. Patients with the less severe OI may have disabilities, but they are not extremely deformed. The two most prominent features of OI are dwarfing and bone fragility. Although a child born today with OI has a better prognosis than a child born thirty or forty years ago, there still has not been a medication discovered that is capable of increasing skeletal structure. The better prognosis results from better general medical care, especially in the treatment of respiratory infections. The younger the child and the more severe the disease, the greater the danger of fracture. Therefore, there is an urgent need for protecting the child. In our case, Basil was a newborn with the more severe form of OI, so our main goal was to protect him.

The child whose limbs are often fractured is a sorry sight. Sometimes parents may be suspected of child abuse when a patient presents multiple or recurring fractures. If the physician considers both OI and child abuse, the diagnosis is usually not difficult. One time our insurance company even questioned us because of the number of claims we had concerning broken bones. Since a diagnosis had already been made, we were cleared of any suspicion. It was certainly an awful feeling to know that anyone even considered abuse as a possibility.

After a diagnosis has been made, the parents need to be educated about the disease. At the time of Basil's birth, not much information was available. Actually, we think that he was the first baby born in Wells County with the severe form of OI.

Today, the physician is more able to answer questions about OI to help the parents know what to expect. In addition, the Osteogenesis Imperfecta Foundation, headquartered in Tampa, Florida, has much information for patients and their families. This information is quite practical because it deals with actually managing the child. The foundation offers a newsletter that focuses on patients, their families, and their accomplishments. The education of the OI child is a major concern. Many OI patients will become productive members of society, and positive education increases their chances for success. These children may benefit academically from being placed in regular classes at school instead of special education classes; however, children with severe cases (like Basil's) cannot be placed in any classroom setting because of the danger of being bumped, as well as the need for individualized attention. Overall, OI patients tend to be above-average in intelligence, and benefit from stimulating environments.

Of all the problems which occur in patients with OI, respiratory infections pose the greatest threat, particularly in those patients who have the severe form of the disease. In newborns, however, the cause of death may be respiratory insufficiency due to inadequate stability of the rib cage. In older children, the major cause of death is respiratory insufficiency due to infection. It seems that the patients with the severe form of OI are in greater jeopardy of this infection since their ribs fracture easily, even with minimal increases in stress. This limits the patients' ability to effectively deal with any type of respiratory infection. These patients also are more likely to have severe rib cage deformities, as well as scoliosis and decreased respiratory capacity. Any respiratory infection, whether upper or lower tract, must be regarded as life-threatening. Sometimes if the patient has a cough, the danger is increased because rib fractures often occur when they cough.

Another concern for OI patients relates to dental problems. The teeth often show abnormalities which lead to progressive erosion of the deciduous teeth and the eventual loss of the permanent teeth. Sometimes the permanent teeth look fairly healthy when they first come in. They may not even deteriorate as rapidly as the baby teeth; however, the basic structure is the same, so similar problems should be expected in time. Basil's permanent teeth appeared to be healthy, but in time, they discolored and seemed to wear down. Good dental care, such as frequent brushing and fluoride treatments, will not cure the problems, but can certainly delay or retard the onset of trouble.

Hearing problems often occur in OI patients. Children under 15 years of age seldom show evidence of hearing loss, but as they enter early adulthood, problems may begin. One of the first signs is the decrease in the ability to hear higher frequencies. Usually nothing can be done to help the OI patient; however, occasionally, a patient may benefit from either a hearing aid or surgical treatment.

One of the biggest problems for Basil was his intolerance of heat. I remember when we drove the van in the winter, most of us would want the heater on. Not Basil! He would ask for the air conditioner to be turned on. Even at home, he was usually warm. We dressed him in light-weight clothing, which helped some. He would still often perspire so much that he would ask for a cold cloth to put on his forehead. Basil also had trouble with constipation, but we were able to control that by adjusting his diet.

Admitting a child with Osteogenesis Imperfecta into a hospital presents many unusual situations for the nursing staff. One of the first things to learn is how to pick up and hold the child. There is little danger of fracturing a bone as long as the head and trunk are supported, as you would do with a normal infant. OI infants cannot tolerate being held more than a few minutes. Even then, you cannot hold them close. Putting the infant on a firm pillow gives support to the entire body which makes the infant more comfortable. I carried Basil on a feather pillow until he was about seven years old. The nursing staff also needs to realize that the body temperature of an OI child tends to be one or two degrees above normal. This may cause dehydration, so water or juice should be offered between feedings.

Parents also face a special set of problems at home with their OI children. Daily tub baths in familiar surroundings are soothing to a child with OI. However, a small tub or basin should be used, and it must be lined with heavy towels or small blankets to cushion the child. For us, it was necessary to add extra counter space to our bathroom vanity so we had a place to put Basil. When he got older, we elevated the bathtub so I did not have to bend over to bathe him; I just leaned against it, which made it much easier to bathe him and to get him in and out. Dressing the OI child can be challenging! The two goals must be comfort for the child and the prevention of fractures. Of course, Basil would say, "And I have to look good, too!"

Light-weight cotton clothing is best because it is absorbent and non-constricting. It is helpful if the clothes open completely down the front or back (especially for infants), and zippers or Velcro closures are preferred to buttons. Changing diapers can be difficult. I had used cloth diapers for Priscilla, and I thought I'd do the same for Basil. But cloth diapers don't slide easily. I was so thankful for the availability of disposable diapers, because they would slide under Basil. I had to lift Basil by placing a hand under his buttocks; if I had lifted him by his ankles, they would have broken. As Basil got older, it was much easier to dress him because he could help me by turning or lifting his legs. Fractures cannot always be prevented. Any sudden jerking motions or turns can cause fracturing. This causes extreme pain for the child. Even the normal routine of getting dressed can cause a fracture. One time we bought Basil a pair of jeans because he wanted to dress like other teens. While I was dressing him, the cuff of the jeans caught on his ankle (his foot turned in) and it broke. I felt awful, but any little thing like that can cause a fracture. Parents also must realize that excessive weight can be a problem. OI children cannot get exercise, so dietary control is necessary.

Approximately 4,000 individuals are afflicted with OI in the United States. These patients face unique medical decisions. The majority are referred to medical centers specializing in this disorder. We usually had to travel to Indianapolis for dental and medical treatment, which was a two-hour drive, one way. Of the 4,000 OI patients, those who have the severe form usually cannot be anesthetized. This is primarily because of the severe respiratory problems which plague these people. We were told that if Basil were ever anesthetized, he would simply never wake up. Even when he had dental surgery and a central line put in, he could not be put to sleep. The doctors told us this when we took Basil to Riley Children's Hospital in Indianapolis to check on a surgical procedure called rodding. This technique is used to straighten the bones of OI children. Because Basil's bones were curved and severely deformed, we decided to find out about rodding. Basil was around seven years old at that time. The doctors felt he was not a good candidate for the surgery because of the danger of not waking up. We had decided not to have the surgery; we wanted Basil to be loved and happy as long as possible. The doctors did show us the X-rays and explained that Basil's bones were so brittle that the rods would have come through the bones, anyway. My husband and I both agreed not to have the surgery because we loved our son too much to take a chance losing him. Since the birth of Basil in 1974, many changes have occurred in the medical profession. One change is in the technique of ultra sound. Today, babies with OI can be diagnosed between the end of the first and the beginning of the second trimester of pregnancy. One of the earliest cases diagnosed was at fourteen weeks. While parents today have the choice of terminating such a pregnancy, we would not have done that to our baby even if we had known about the OI. I can understand the viewpoint of parents who may choose to terminate the pregnancy because they feel they cannot deal with such a challenging situation. Parents must be willing to face additional stress in the family, extra medical bills, and the continuous care of an OI child. However, if I had known about Basil and his OI, I would still have wanted him. I do not regret one moment of my time spent with Basil.

As we left the hospital with our baby in March of 1974, I was shouldered with one additional burden. The doctors, and probably all the medical personnel, believed and told us that Basil probably would not survive his first few weeks.

BASIL'S HOMECOMING

On that cold, windy day as Basil left the hospital with his nervous and apprehensive parents, I remember thinking, "What am I going to do? Now I'm on my own." I had never seen him bathed, and had only seen him dressed once. Part of the problem was that only the head nurse gave Basil care while in the hospital; and I know that she was terrified of someone else (or even herself) breaking his bones. I guess she really didn't know what to tell me about caring for him. She carried him out to the car on a pillow that Basil Sr. had brought to the hospital. On the way home, I told my husband that I hoped I could handle this. At twenty-four years of age, I could only pray that I had the common sense and ability to do what had to be done so our son could survive.

When we arrived home, both grandmas and Priscilla were anxiously waiting for us. It was very obvious that we all were nervous about this fragile little baby. I remember how we all passed Priscilla around the day she came home from the hospital. I also remember how thrilled I was with my first child. I dressed her up in practically every outfit she had! Both of my kids had full heads of long, black hair. I brushed Priscilla's hair and tried out all of her hair bows and barrettes. What fun! But this time things were different. Even the grandmas were too afraid to hold their newest grandchild. I was worried about even changing his clothes or diapers when needed; I didn't even think about trying different clothes on him. I was even afraid to bathe him and wash his hair. Instead of the homecoming being a joyous time for our family, it was one of stress and awkwardness.

Part of the awkwardness was because Basil Sr. had not told any of our families, friends, or fellow workers that anything was wrong with our son. He was, I suppose, keeping all of his thoughts and worries to himself. Even though I had known during my pregnancy that something was wrong, Basil (as well as the doctors) thought I was just worrying over nothing. I was not surprised when they finally told me about Basil's condition; however, my husband was not really prepared because he truly believed that nothing could go wrong. My husband deals with stress and problems by burying himself in continuous work. He's not one to talk out his problems, but he sure knows how to "work" them out. But our families and friends understood this about him. They were not upset that he had kept our baby's serious condition from them. Rather, they were worried about how Basil Sr. was handling the situation.

The only thing that changed for me once I knew something was wrong with my baby was the name I had chosen for him. Because my pregnancy had been so difficult, I knew I would not be able to have any more children. At first, I had picked out the name "Christopher Lee" for a boy. When Basil Jr. was born, I knew that he was the only son we would ever have. I also knew that I really wanted to name him after his daddy. So, we had Basil Sr. and Basil Jr. I know this meant a great deal to my husband, and still does. Even when Basil carried our son into our home for the first time, we could tell how proud he was of his little boy. No father could have loved his son any more, but I was the one who had to learn how to care for our new baby. That job fell to me.

And so there we were. I knew I could not wait any longer. My baby had been home two days, and it was time for his first bath at home. It was awful. I had to sit down and think it through before I could even start. I decided to make a little bed of towels on the counter beside the sink. I scooted his little head over the edge of the sink and shampooed his hair. Then I gently scooted him back on the towels and washed him. Mom was there, so as I held him, she washed his back. The whole process took most of an hour. By the time he was six months old, I felt confident enough to put him in one of those baby bathtubs. I still lined the bottom with layers of towels, but it sure made the bathing process much easier. We used this tub until he was about four years old. By then, Basil Sr. had built up our regular bathtub at home.

Feeding our baby presented its own special problems. Because he was so small, I had to feed him smaller amounts, but more frequently. He seemed to have trouble digesting milk, so we used Jell-o water a lot. When he was about four weeks old, he lost weight and was down to just over four pounds. This added to the doctors' belief that Basil probably would not live. There wasn't any specific thing we could do; I just kept feeding him and loving him. With time, he slowly gained back his birth weight. Of course, we did not want him to ever get overweight because of his small stature. Even at age eighteen, his peak weight was around 27 pounds.

Priscilla's reaction to her new brother was very normal. She wanted to kiss him and touch him and hold him. I was terrified at first that she would hurt him. I always worried that she would tip over his bassinet as she stood at the side, peering at her little "Bubby." But I talked with her and explained how fragile her little brother was. She seemed to understand, and we just worked with her so she could learn what she could and could not do. Because it took so much of my time to care for Basil, I often worried about not spending enough time with Priscilla. Again, my mom helped out. She tried to do things with Priscilla to make her feel special. I'll always appreciate the support Mom gave to us. For the first year, I was the only one to really care for Basil. Basil Sr. was working most of the time, and nobody else felt like they could handle Junior without hurting him. Mom and Frank were good about doing my grocery shopping for me. I remember one of the doctors telling me that Basil Sr. and I should get away together, if only just to grab a hamburger. But there never seemed to be time.

Usually, parents welcome visitors when they have a new baby. We, too, were glad for the support of our families and friends. However, we rarely got any sleep during those first two years. Basil slept very little, and cried most of his waking moments. Basil Sr. and I took turns holding our baby on a pillow and rocking him for hours. Sometimes he would go to sleep, and we would ease him, pillow and all, into his crib. We would tiptoe quietly into bed, and maybe get to sleep for a few minutes, and then the crying would begin again. Very few people realize the amount of stress that put on our family. We had to sleep whenever we could; sometimes I would not even answer the door if one of us was resting. Even though we were exhausted most of the time, we never argued. Somehow God gave us the strength to meet our challenge and still care for each other. The fact that our son had this disease was really never an issue which divided us. We simply loved him, and tried to do our very best for him, and for each other.

BASIL'S EARLY YEARS

When Bubby was a little over a year old, we decided I would go back to work at Corning. I wasn't sure if I could manage both responsibilities, but Basil told me to just try it, and if it didn't work, I would quit. The people at Corning were so good to me. They had allowed me to take a leave of absence after Bubby was born so I didn't have to actually quit. We both worked at Corning, and we worked the same shift. The first consideration was who would stay with Bubby while we were at work. Mom volunteered to help us out; at the time, she worked days, so she could stay with Bubby while we were at work. She spent many hours rocking him to quiet him down. It wasn't that Bubby was a bad baby, but just that he was always in so much pain. One time, Mom's shift was changed at work, and we needed a new sitter. My friend, Cheryl, volunteered to help out. She had her own kids, as well as one child for whom she babysat. We took Bubby to her house since it was on our way to work. After about the second night, she realized what his life was like. I remember what she said to me after that night. "How can you do this and work? I've rocked him, held him, given him a bottle—nothing helped. He still cried all night." I told her that I was getting used to it, and I just managed somehow. Shortly after that, Mom was able to trade shifts so she could babysit for Bubby again.

We had a few people we trusted to care for him, but sometimes everyone would be busy. One time we needed a sitter so we could go to work. I hired a girl who had been told of Bubby's special needs. I was working the earlier evening shift, so I called home to check on Basil Jr. I got a busy signal, so I tried again later. That phone was busy the entire time! I decided to call our neighbor and ask him to go check on Basil and the sitter.

He chose to walk over to Bubby's bedroom window to listen, and he heard Bubby crying. He went back home so I could call him. When he told me what was going on, I was furious. My shift was ending, so I was able to get home quickly. She was off the phone by the time we got home, and she was ready to leave. I asked her how things had gone, thinking maybe she would be honest. Instead, she told me that he went to sleep early and had been resting fine. She left, and I went back to his room to check on him. His door had been completely closed, but when I opened the door, the room reeked of vomit. I was mortified! He had vomited from crying so hard and eventually fell asleep. I had to wake him up, and give him a bath, as well as change his bed. I was so thankful he didn't choke. That girl never sat for us again. I still get upset when I think of this incident today. We fought to keep our son alive, and it could have all ended in just a few minutes because of someone's negligence.

After that, we decided that if we could not work out the babysitting among family, I simply would not work. We were able to work out some sort of schedule, crazy as it was to get, and I was able to stay at Corning four years.

Just as one would do with normal children, we wanted to help Basil become as independent as he could. He learned to talk very easily, probably because he was around adults most of the time. His tongue was a little large for his mouth, and he had a tendency to speak quickly. Other than that, his speech developed normally, and by two years of age, he was speaking well. I guess I didn't rush into teaching him to feed himself or anything else until I felt he was strong enough. When he was very young, Priscilla played little games with Bubby. One time they were playing in the bedroom when I heard him crying. I checked on them, and Priscilla had placed a single sheet of paper on his face in a kind of hide-and-seek game. He simply could not get the paper off of his face, and was crying. Then I realized just how weak he really was. As he became older, he developed more strength. When he was nearly three years old, I tried letting him hold his own food. At first, I let him hold a fourth of a jelly sandwich. After getting used to the coordination of putting that little sandwich in his mouth, he was able to do that without much of a mess.

I began to realize how important it would be as years went along for Bubby to do some things for himself. Even though I knew he could not do a lot, I believed he could accomplish some tasks—and it was necessary for his own self-esteem. So I decided to help him learn to feed himself completely. Since he was flat on his back all the time, I had to use a small pillow to prop him up a bit. I turned him on his side a little, and that's the position we used for eating the rest of his life. At first, I filled his spoon for him, and then he took it and ate. Once he mastered that, I propped his bowl up, and let him dip the spoon into the bowl. Basil loved this little bit of independence, but it was very hard for Grandma Sarah (my mom) to accept. "Dorothy Jean, why do you have that baby feeding himself?" I guess Mom thought I was pushing him too hard, but he loved it. Once he learned, he refused to let anyone feed him. Of course, when he had a broken arm, I would have to help him; other than that, he fed himself. He drank with a straw. He learned to balance a glass by using his body. We seldom used a glass with a lid, so he really got pretty good at handling glasses full of beverages. He kept a glass of iced tea with him nearly all the time.

Bubby had been feeding himself for about a year, and he was four years old. I decided it was silly to let him potty in a diaper, since he had a good mind and he knew when he had to go. So one day I told him that it was kind of foolish to be spending so much money on diapers when I knew he was old enough to be trained. He agreed with me. We decided to forget the diapers, and he would tell me when he had to go. If he had to urinate, I would hold a cup for him to go in. If he needed to have a bowel movement, then I'd put a diaper on so he could go. The first couple times he used the "pee cup" he almost wet his pants. But he soon remembered he had no diaper on, so then it was OK. This potty training only took about one day! It was normal for others to treat Basil like a baby because of his size and limitations. So I felt it was vital to make him feel more like a four-year-old. He seemed to take pride in being able to master some of these "normal" tasks.

Parents worry about how to discipline their children. With Priscilla, I believed a good swat on the bottom was needed from time to time. However, Bubby was different. I know people find it hard to believe that someone like Basil would even need to be disciplined. But he did. Even though I only had to discipline him five or six times, I felt he needed to know the limits. I used a flyswatter, and just lightly brushed across his little leg. I knew it didn't actually hurt anything except his feelings. But that was effective. His main problem was arguing with me. He always liked being clean and tidy. One time I had just cleaned him up and given him his lunch. He had one of his jelly sandwiches, and a drop of jelly fell onto his pillowcase. He wanted the pillowcase changed immediately. Well, everything had been clean to start with, so I took a damp cloth and washed the jelly off. He insisted that wasn't good enough. I explained that it was all cleaned off, and it was nothing to worry about. His dark eyes snapped, and he said, "If I could only get to that phone, I'd call the cops and get you for child abuse." It was kind of funny, but I didn't dare laugh because he was so serious. Later on, we both were able to laugh about it.

Bubby loved going to Grandma Sarah's house, which he started doing when he was three years old. The reason he liked it so much is that Mom and Frank (Mom's husband and Basil's grandpa) devoted the entire day to him. Frank would sit at the table with Basil and play a game of catch. Basil tossed a ping pong ball to Frank, and Frank would catch it in a bowl. He'd give it back to Bubby, and they'd do it all over again. Frank played this for hours with him. He was so willing to spend time with Basil just because he loved him. As Basil got older, they played Rook, Rummy, checkers, and other games sometimes even until late at night. Mom often played the games with Frank and Basil. She also bathed him, dressed him, and cooked for him. Like all grandmas, she enjoyed fixing the special food that he liked. Although he dearly loved spending the night with Grandma and Frank, he would always call me several times. He'd want to know what I was doing, or what time I got up, or what I was eating. He especially wanted to know my plans for the day; I guess he didn't want to miss out on anything!

One significant event at about this time was our decision to move from town to the country. Priscilla was six years old, and Bubby was four. We thought we wanted quieter surroundings, and I didn't want to have the worry of Priscilla wanting to wander off with neighbor kids to the park. I guess I had enough to deal with, and I didn't need that extra worry. Basil Sr. built a new house for us, and as soon as we moved, we realized that it was the best thing we could have done. Two nearby neighbors built their houses at about the same time, so we all became friends. Priscilla could play on the patio or in the yard, and I didn't have to worry. We had good neighbors. Just to the east of us were Mike and Deb Johns with their two boys, Jeremy, age two, and Brady, about five or six months old. Eventually we all became good friends; the boys were buddies to Basil, and we even ended up trading houses later on. Our other neighbors were Emil and Ellen Breedlove. They were good neighbors to have, and always willing to help us out. Ellen stayed with Bubby once in a while if I needed to go get medicine or run some other errand. Having had such good neighbors smoothed our way.

One Picture

Is Worth A

Thousand Words

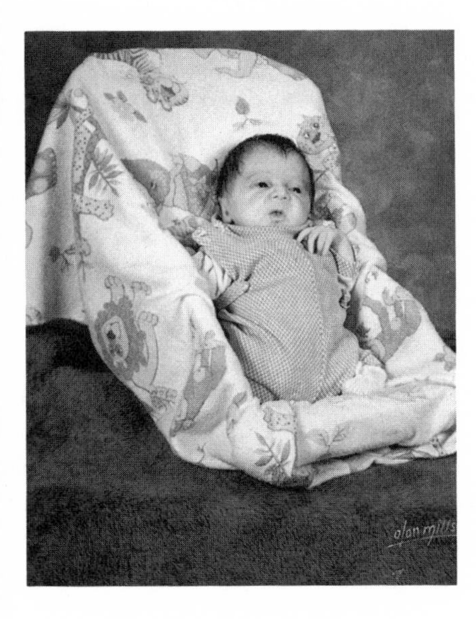

Our new son:
age three weeks.

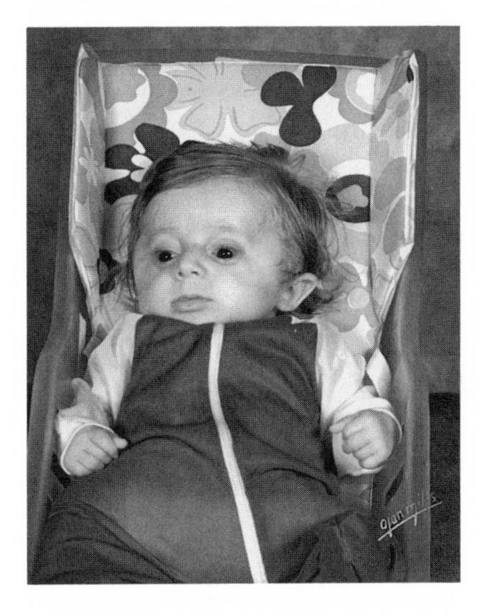

Basil age two years.

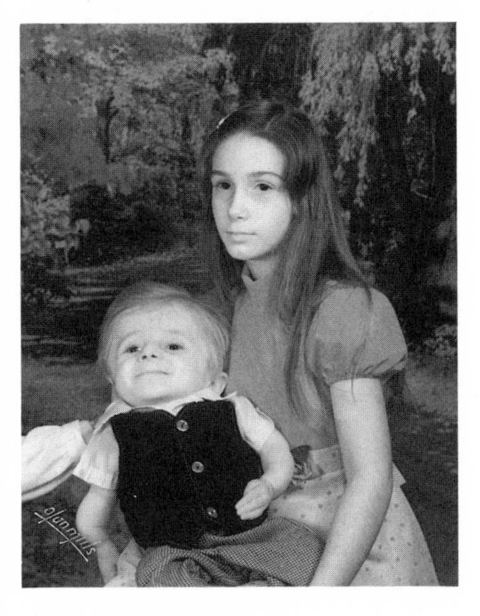

Priscilla was 10 and Basil 7
when this photo was taken.

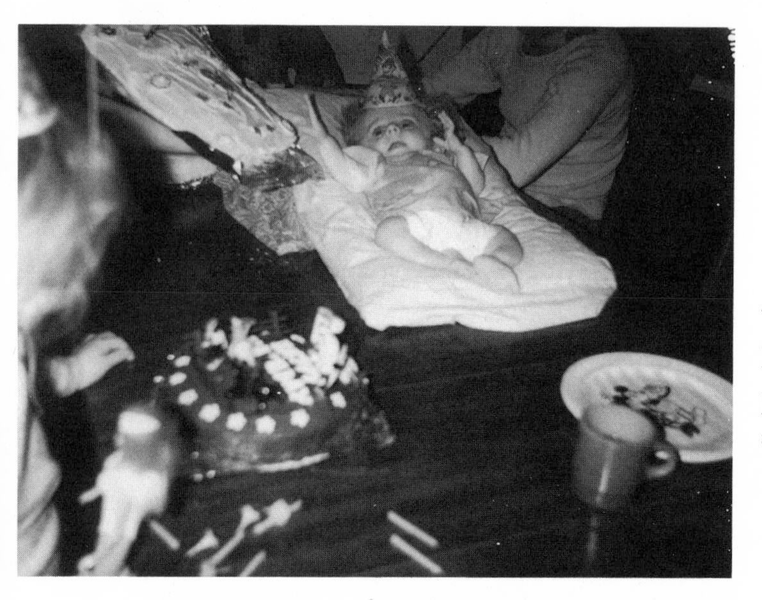

The Rhodes kids had their birthday party together, at age 2 and 5.

Basil's 3rd birthday party was at McDonald's with family and friends.

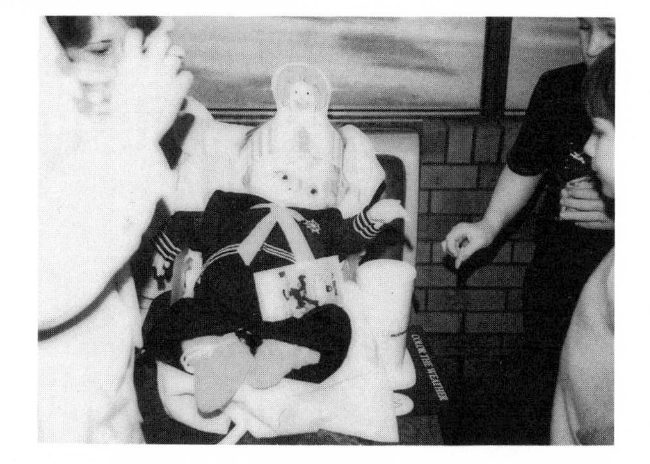

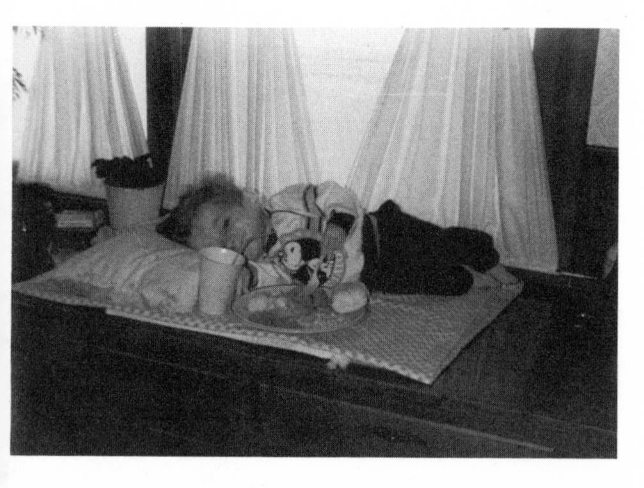

This hearty eater's favorite meal was beef and noodles with mashed potatoes, corn, baked beans, hot rolls, and iced tea.

SCHOOL DAYS

Now that Basil was nearing school age, we had some important decisions to make. We knew the value of a good education, and we wanted the best for our son. Education of the handicapped student can sometimes be a delicate situation. We had read that; surely the OI foundation talked about educating these often bright children as a priority. We decided to start with pre-school. Because Basil was homebound, it was necessary for the teacher to come to our home. The first step was to have him tested by special services. These test results ended up causing us a lot of grief. Basil was tested August 9, 1978, in our home. The following information is from the clinician's report:

BEHAVIOR OBSERVATIONS

As stated it was necessary to visit the home of Basil Rhodes in order to perform psychological testing. It was rated Basil is a verbal, seemingly bright, curious, and responsive child with clear speech. He was a friendly and cooperative child, and is obviously hampered on performing any test items that will involve any motor skills. He seemed emotionally intact and content in his home; and appeared remarkably well-adjusted considering the pervasiveness of the disease process. Basil's test results on the Slossan Intelligence Test, his mental age of three years yielded an I.Q. of 67. Basil failed items beginning at four month level all the way through the five year level that required any muscular-skeletal skills. He was unable to complete any item that involved neuro-muscular. His verbal skills are developed in an age appropriate manner, so his

> *I.Q. score is lower than his verbal abilities. On the Peabody Picture Vocabulary Test the examiner observed it was difficult for Basil to make clear the picture he was pointing at. Which again he was trying to use muscular-skeletal skills.*

The "Summaries, Conclusions, and Recommendations" of this report is probably one of the saddest ever reviewed by a parent.

> *Basil was seen, tested and found to be functioning in the Mild Range of mental retardation. His verbal skills, general knowledge and information, auditory memory, knowledge of body parts, arithmetic reasoning, knowledge of common objects in the environment, and other verbally related skills appear to be developed within an age appropriate fashion.*

First of all, we were angry that our obviously bright son was labeled as "mildly retarded." Furthermore, I want it to be known that this lady only met Basil and our family the day of the testing. But yet she had the nerve to recommend that in the interest of the mental health of the family, consideration should be given to eventual alternative care. She believed that the family, over a period of time, should prepare themselves to place Basil in a setting where he could receive alternative care and where the family could begin to live a more "normal lifestyle."

It's very difficult for me to understand how the lady who gave Basil this test arrived at these scores and opinions of how our lifestyle was. She stated Basil was content and well-adjusted in his home. It was also mentioned in the report that Basil was obviously hampered on performing any test involving motor skills, but he was still tested on these skills and evaluated on the outcomes. Apparently she forgot to mention at the time of the testing that Basil's left arm was broken! I feel this report should have been reviewed by the school much more closely and not accepted into Basil's permanent records. The test was a total disadvantage to my son and I should have spoken out at the time to refuse permission for the testing because it was an inappropriate test for a child with limited motor skills. I really regret that I've waited so long to speak out about this. It is wrong that someone from a school system could come into our home for a couple of hours, leave, and then write a callous and damaging report which would change our already satisfactory life into a nightmare for all of us. I'd like very much to let everyone know that I did everything possible to see that my son had all the love and care he needed both day and night.

At home, my family and I felt we had a lifestyle that was wonderful and unique, especially with Basil Jr., with the terrific times together, and a strong love that we all shared as a family. It took ten years of my asking to get this distorted and inaccurate evaluation of my son's I.Q. out of his school records. Finally, I had to hire a lawyer who charged me three hundred dollars for a trip to the school in order to go through Basil's files. Why did we have to go to the expense and hassle of hiring a lawyer and put ourselves through such mental anguish? Once my lawyer went to the school, the results of Basil's test and evaluation were removed from his file and given to me by the school.

Basil's formal education started with preschool. His teacher came to our house twice a week for about two hours each time. They worked on the usual preschool subjects, like using blocks to develop motor skills. These early years were rough for Bubby because his body was still so fragile. In spite of the fact that his bones broke frequently, sometimes necessitating decreasing instructional hours because of his pain, he still managed to pick up the necessary skills.

His life and growth as a person continued. Because he was so delicate, Basil spent most of his time at home, except when we would travel to West Virginia to visit family. Relatives often visited us and would talk to Bubby, and, of course, play cards. (All Grandpa Rhodes and Bubby wanted to play was Rook!) Uncle Gary and his boys, Phillip and Danny, often talked sports with Basil. Maybe that's how he became such a sports fanatic, even at such a young age. His interest in Indiana University basketball and the New York Mets baseball team probably began during this time.

Before we knew it, the time had come for kindergarten. Sometimes unforeseen problems come up for homebound students. Basil's kindergarten teacher actually taught at the high school half days, and then spent an afternoon twice a week with Bubby. After about four weeks of school, I was aware he seemed bored with class. I decided to take him to school for class with the other children, hoping that would spark his interest. They were working on telling time, and other things that were more difficult than what Basil had been working on with the homebound teacher. As soon as I told his teacher the kinds of activities his class was doing, she began working on those exact lessons the next day. She didn't realize the level of difficulty kindergarteners could handle. We learned a couple of things from this experience. First, if a tutor does not keep in close contact with the classroom teacher, it is difficult to keep up with the students in school. Secondly, if the teacher doesn't normally teach children close to the same age, she's lost in preparing lessons for a homebound student.

Basil was a very bright student who was eager to learn. From first through the eighth grades, Basil had some very special teachers who realized he was one who always had to achieve well or he wasn't satisfied with himself at all. He was always upset with himself when he scored less than perfect; he was even angry with himself if his score fell into the "B" range. After many discussions about this perfectionism, Basil Jr. decided to be more tolerant of his less-than-perfect grades. He even managed to jokingly try to bribe his teachers to get a grade changed! Of course, that approach did not work, but it shows how wonderfully Basil wove his sense of humor into his daily life.

Basil received five hours of schooling a week through the eighth grade. I can remember many special moments from those years. During this time, Jeremy and Brady Johns started coming over for short visits. At first it was somewhat awkward, until everyone became comfortable. Deb used to worry that the boys would stay too long and tire Basil out. We soon learned that a very special friendship was developing. At first, the boys would watch cartoons with Bubby; then they would talk about everything. Once Jeremy and Brady became used to Basil and his limitations, they all but refused to accept those limitations. They always tried to figure out some way of including Basil in what they were doing. A special baseball game was created just for Basil. Using a ping pong ball for the baseball, a pencil for the bat, and pillows for the bases, the boys played ball! This was an inside game, usually played in the winter, and the boys ran bases for Basil. They all took turns batting. This was a great way for Bubby to enjoy himself. Playing ball was a normal, everyday activity for the boys; for Basil, it was a major accomplishment to be a part of such a normal activity. In the summer, one of their favorite games was Cowboys and Indians—using squirt guns, of course. The boys rigged up one of the guns somehow so that Basil could actually squirt out the water. He could not pull the trigger because he didn't have the strength. Using a clothes pin, and I don't know what else, they adapted that gun so he could squirt it. Basil didn't get to do that a lot because of the weather and his health, but he sure enjoyed the days he did. As all three boys got older, they became interested in video games. Starting with Atari, the boys upgraded their game playing with Nintendo, and then computer games. The hours they spent playing those games! I can still hear that music to "Frogger" in my mind. Often Jeremy and Brady would spend the night here. They played games until late at night; first thing the next morning, the games started again. What great fun they all had!

When Basil was in fifth grade, Sally Shively became his teacher, and she was an outstanding one. She came to the house for class, or sometimes I would take him into school. Sally always made him feel a part of her class at school. The students considered Basil one of their classmates. One time Basil really wanted me to leave him there alone. I was nervous about that; I trusted Sally, but I knew how children swarmed around Basil. But I decided to try it; he had a wonderful time, and nothing dangerous happened. Our local radio station sponsored a special teacher recognition. Basil decided to submit Mrs. Shively's name, and her name was mentioned on the radio. Of course, Bubby had to send her roses in honor of the occasion! Mrs. Shively had her turn to surprise Basil on his eleventh birthday, March 4, 1985. We had planned Basil would visit school that day. The whole class had planned a birthday party, complete with balloons and a special cake. Mrs. Shively always referred to her classes as

"Shively's Sharpies" and Basil was one of them. The kids gave Basil a heart-shaped pillow on which they had signed their names. They also made a little card tree for all of his birthday cards. Basil remembered that day as one of his favorite times.

During the middle school years, kids often become very concerned with their peers' opinions of them. Basil was no exception. We were forced to trade cars when Corning shut down and Basil Sr. was laid off. He went to a car auction in West Virginia and sold our Cadillac and bought an older car; actually, what he bought was a clunker! It had been snowing, so Basil really couldn't see all of the car's body. After he bought it, he discovered that it was a blue car, but it had a red hood. When Bubby found out, he was mortified. I had to take him to school in it one day, and he insisted that I park around to the side and put him in his stroller. He said, "Mom, I don't want to be caught in this old clunker!" I guess he really wasn't so different, after all.

Another special memory from middle school was bitter-sweet. Because Basil was a good speller, he became a candidate for the class spelling bee. He practiced a lot, and felt ready for the challenge. Basil was excited when we arrived at school for the bee. However, maybe he was too excited, because he misspelled the very first word. All of the other students wanted to give him another chance. But I said no, because I wanted him to be treated like all the other kids his age. Nobody else would have been given a second chance, so I didn't think he should have one, either. He cried because he was so disappointed. I tried to explain to him that it had been a different experience for him because this time he wasn't the only student; he was competing with others and he was probably affected by the extra pressure. Even though he was greatly disappointed, he never questioned my judgment.

The following year Basil became a freshman at Bluffton High School. At the beginning of that year, we learned that by state law he should have received four hours a day of instruction starting in the seventh grade. Actually, he had only received five hours a week during those two years. The school system was simply unaware of this law since Basil was the first permanently homebound student in the corporation. As a parent, I was certainly not knowledgeable about the laws. My reaction was one of frustration and a feeling that my son had been cheated in his education. However, even though his hours in junior high were fewer than they should have been, Basil still entered with excellent preparation and work. Obviously he had not been hurt by this oversight. I was able to accept the situation as long as it would be corrected.

The longer hours for Basil in school were much more difficult than they would have been for a healthy student. But he had such a will to learn and to try new things, he actually handled the extra hours well. Basil said, "All a person has to do is get interested in his subjects and the time passes fast."

But as we all know, the teacher has to make the discussions interesting, also. Basil did get the extra time in class, but he became so flustered with his freshman year during the first few weeks of school that I was concerned about how class was being conducted. Always before, Basil had class in his bedroom. But at the conference for his freshman year, it was decided that it would be better for him if he had more involvement with the classroom. So, the school videotaped the classes to which Basil was assigned. Our VCR was in the living room so that's where Basil Jr. had class. When I realized there was a problem in class I began to listen in on how the tapes were being used. The teacher was trying to teach Basil primarily from the tapes. All afternoon the VCR was on and off, making a loud roaring noise that would make anyone lose interest in what was being studied. Basil had plenty of homework to do but he was having trouble understanding it. That had never been a problem before. It seemed I was doing the teacher's work in the evenings. I became as frustrated as Basil; besides, it was too long a day with all the unnecessary homework left for him to do in the evenings.

I called Basil's school to express my concern; a conference was scheduled. I explained how the tapes were being used. I also mentioned spending every evening doing homework with Basil that he didn't understand. It wasn't that I minded helping my son; he was a joy to me in everything we did together. I felt the teacher should be spending time explaining the concepts to Basil so that he could do his work. Apparently the teacher wasn't willing to change her techniques; she declined to continue teaching him.

It was approximately three weeks before she was replaced with a wonderful teacher named Deb Johnson. Deb appeared on the first day with a big smile on her face. From then on, Basil and Deb enjoyed every school day they had together. She was patient and explained everything until he understood it completely. Every morning he was awake by 7:15 and ready for breakfast. Then I'd dress him for class, comb his hair, and let him brush his teeth. Basil was always anxious for Deb to get there so they could get started for the day. He always had a big smile to greet her with, himself, and usually had something funny to say when she entered his room. God works in unique and special ways. After spending a few weeks together, Basil and Deb became convinced that God brought them together.

I think I agreed. Evelyn Priddy was responsible for getting a teacher for Basil. Evelyn worked for the school system, but didn't really know Deb. Deb was a licensed English and reading teacher, but was staying at home with her two children. The spring before Basil needed a teacher, Deb had volunteered to help with kindergarten round-up at the elementary school. This was the first time she had ever done that; it was also the responsibility of Evelyn Priddy to organize and supervise the round-up procedure. Later that summer, looking for an apartment, Evelyn telephoned "the Johnsons" whom she had heard were managers of an apartment complex in town. Unknown to Evelyn, Deb Johnson and her husband, Dave, were those managers. Evelyn ended up moving into the apartment complex, and all of these events set the stage for Evelyn when she needed a new teacher for Basil. Evelyn and Deb became better acquainted through the manager-tenant relationship. Just a few weeks after Evelyn moved in, she contacted Deb about a possible part-time teaching position. In Basil's and Deb's minds, these events were all guided by God to bring the two of them together. Because the relationship between Basil and Deb was so deep and exceptional, affecting all of our lives, I want her to tell her part of the story in her own words.

Dear Dorothy,

I would be delighted to talk about my favorite student! When Evelyn Priddy first contacted me about teaching a homebound student, I had some reservations. First, I had two children, and one was not yet in school. I knew I wanted to eventually get back into full-time teaching, but I wasn't quite ready for that. Since this was a part-time teaching position, however, it was appealing. My second reservation was that I had never worked with a student who had severe physical limitations. I asked Evelyn if she would be able to meet with me to discuss teaching Basil; over a cup of tea, we discussed his strong academic abilities as well as his extremely limited physical abilities. My primary question was "What if I'm not the kind of teacher Basil needs?" We agreed that I would try, and if it didn't work, Evelyn would continue looking for a teacher. Well, she didn't have to look again!

My first impression of Basil was one of awe and compassion. I was amazed at his natural curiosity, his quick sense of humor, and his perseverance. And, yes, I was touched—touched by not only his physical limitations, but also the pain he endured nearly every moment of his life. At first I worried about feeling pity for him. I knew I could not allow that to interfere in our student-teacher relationship. I shouldn't have worried, though—Basil didn't let anyone feel sorry for him. Sympathy and empathy, perhaps, but never pity. Basil and I knew we were a team right from the start. I knew he had been struggling with his schoolwork that year. He had been behind in a class or two, and that really upset Basil. Because he was so discouraged, I decided to give him an upbeat nickname. I nicknamed Basil "Maestro." He truly was a maestro of life. Basil had a gift for enjoying life in spite of his constant pain and discomfort. We spent four to five hours a day together. I taught all of the subjects, except for computer. We worked with the high school teachers so Basil and I would cover the same material as other students in his class. Basil needed periodic breaks, just as all high school students do. At the end of each subject, we would take a short break. One time during the morning we would take a longer break so Basil could have a snack. Those breaks became our time to just enjoy our friendship. We would have a snack together while listening to one of Basil's many Christian rock tapes. During this time we would catch up on the lives of our families. Over the two years that I taught Basil, I became friends with his family. Basil Sr., Dorothy, and Priscilla were always a most loving support group for Basil. The four of them were very close, especially Maestro and his mother. Dorothy was the primary caregiver for Basil, and they had a wonderful, positive relationship. Teaching Basil was a joy! It is the highlight of my teaching career. He continually challenged me with his intelligent questions. I learned a lot about subjects I had not studied in years. Although my license is in English and reading, I also taught algebra, history, science, health, or whatever subjects Basil chose to take. Every day was exciting for us because we both learned. It was a challenge for me to come up with new ways to explain concepts. Usually it was the little things that were the most difficult. For example, Basil always had to be in a reclining position, either on his back or side. His perspective when riding in their van was quite different from my perspective. If I talked about a new store that was north of town by a grocery store, he most likely would not be able to relate to my directions. Since he couldn't see out of the van windows, he did not know the landmarks. Another time he was taking a test where he had to identify pictures. On one picture, Basil was very puzzled. "Is this a broom?" he finally guessed. "It has a long handle." As I explained to him that it was actually a rake, I realized that he probably had never seen a rake before, at least not up close. It was then that I began to understand how limited Basil's experiences necessarily were, because of his handicap.

One of the lessons that was the most fun was in a health chapter on physical fitness. Basil had no idea what it meant to do the exercises mentioned in the chapter. I decided to wear my sweats one day and I showed him how to do the exercises. I took the fit-

ness test in the chapter, and he counted and timed me. I excelled in one area, but miserably failed in another! It was entertaining, but Basil also had a first hand experience of what those exercises were like. Of course, he teased me a lot about that one failed test! Our biology teacher loaned me a special microscope that turned in such a way that enabled Basil to see through it. Dorothy would put him on the table with one of his prop pillows, and then we would set up the microscope. Other than poking Basil in the eye one time, I managed it OK! It was a marvelous experience for him to be able to see the same kinds of things his classmates did. Basil was so patient with me as I learned the best methods of teaching him. During our freshman year, I often would forget and hold papers in a way that he couldn't see them clearly. "I can't see that, Deb," he gently reminded me.

We soon adjusted to each other so well that we could anticipate each others' words and thoughts. The unusual aspect of our relationship was that it was one-on-one for up to five hours a day. How rare for one person to have that kind of quality time with another person! I consider it a privilege to have spent that time with Maestro. Basil had the gift of turning any day into sunshine. No matter what state of mind I would be in, I was always in a more positive, uplifted mood when I left. Basil and I were more than just student and teacher; we were friends, and I loved him. Basil's sense of humor was contagious. He had such a clever wit about him, and he delighted in using puns as well as vocabulary words. One of Basil's joys was to throw out a computer term during class, knowing that I was basically computer illiterate! However, he also interjected our English vocabulary words into his computer class conversation to "test" his teacher, Evelyn Priddy. He was invariably correct in his usage. Of course, being a true Indiana University fan, we had endless jokes about any team that played IU. He attempted to teach me about IU players, chess, and computers. The teaching role satisfied Basil so much that I even allowed him to be the teacher for a day. He would prepare the lesson and quiz me;

however, he could only do that when he was feeling good and that was not very often.

A special aspect of our relationship was a spiritual one. After being together for just a few days, we realized that we were indeed a team. We both believed the circumstances that brought us together were more than just circumstances. No one could convince us that God had not brought us together intentionally. We often talked about God, and what it means to be a Christian. Prayer became just one more bond between us. As Basil's condition worsened, we prayed together more frequently. I remember one day when the Make-A-Wish Foundation had called. Dorothy mentioned this to Basil during break, stating that he would need to decide what wish to request. After our break, I noticed that Basil seemed a little preoccupied. When I asked him if anything was wrong, he replied, "Wishes don't come true, anyway." I pursued the comment by asking him what he would wish for. He answered that he wished he could walk and play baseball. With tear-filled eyes, I responded that I knew his wish probably would not come true in this life, but that I knew God had a baseball waiting for Basil in heaven. And I believe that today Basil is whole.

When we had to stop Basil's schooling in late October of 1990, my world literally fell apart. Although Dorothy had mentioned throughout the summer that he was not as strong as he had been, I guess I just refused to accept reality. It did happen abruptly. One day during class, he suddenly cried out and raised his tiny hands to hold his head. Several bones had "popped"—broken or moved—in his head. His pain was more intense and constant than it had ever been. It never lessened. That was our last day of class.

In a way, ending our special relationship was like a death to me. Even though his family and friends still had Basil in their lives, I did not. I continued to visit him both in the hospital and at home, but it wasn't the same. As I look back, I realize that I was actually in mourning. I couldn't concentrate on anything; I forgot responsibilities, and I was depressed. To make matters worse, I had to begin substitute teaching in order to continue helping out financially at home. Many days I found myself in tears, not wanting to even leave the house, but forcing myself to go through the routine of daily life. One evening Evelyn Priddy phoned to see how Basil was doing. As I talked with her, I began to cry. I shared how lost I felt, and frustrated that I wasn't able to take control of my emotions. It was Evelyn who suggested that I was probably mourning the abrupt absence of Basil from my life. Once I could understand why I was feeling that way, I could begin to deal with those feelings. And I did. Starting that evening after my talk with Evelyn, I tried talking with my family more about my feelings. My husband was surprised to realize the impact this situation had on me. My in-laws were visiting that night, and as I explained the phone call from Evelyn, I again began sobbing. My wonderful mother-in-law took me in her arms and let me cry. Then I was able to share the intensity of my loss. And that began the slow process of my healing.

How was my life changed since Basil became a part of it? I'm a richer, more complete person and teacher. I think I've learned to be more content with my life, and to appreciate each separate goodness in life, no matter how small. Basil also taught me to love life enough to persevere through times of pain or difficulty. His faith grew, and I found it inspiring that he could remain faithful to God in spite of the terrible pain and discomfort he experienced.

And so, Basil, I want you to know you've been a special part of my life, and I love you. Someday, we'll be singing praises to God together again; and, Maestro, how about a game of catch?

I'm thankful Deb shared her own experiences with Basil. We still keep in touch quite a bit since we live in the same community, and have developed a strong friendship. Working on this book has been a welcome release for both of us.

As Deb has said, her time with Basil came to an abrupt end in the fall of his high school junior year, 1990. The summer of 1990 had not been a good one for Basil. His head hurt him nearly all the time. I sensed he just wasn't himself. He seemed rather depressed; I was the only one who noticed it, though. Of course, Bubby had a real talent for hiding the way he felt, especially in front of friends and relatives. The doctor had already prescribed Tylenol with codeine for his severe headaches; however, she soon had to prescribe morphine by mouth, and then finally methadone pills. Nothing relieved his pain. Even today we are not certain what caused his terrible pain. Some doctors believed it might be related to nerve problems in his head; others thought there was an enormous amount of pressure on his brain. One doctor even considered the possibility of an aneurism. Finally the pain and the powerful medicine were too much for Basil. I know he was really worried about starting up school in August. His concern was mainly that he would not feel good enough to do well in his classes. We even talked about quitting, but he just didn't want to give up on his education. After talking it over with us and Deb, he decided to start the school year, and take one day at a time. Those days lasted only about six weeks; Basil's head popped badly one day in class, and things seemed to get worse after that. In mid-October, Basil had to quit his schooling. Even though he hurt all the time, he was disappointed that he had not been able to earn his high school diploma.

I talked with Deb frequently about Basil's health. We both knew how important that high school diploma was to him. Deb talked to the school superintendent about the possibility of getting Basil a diploma, even if it was an honorary one. He seemed to support the idea, but nothing was actually decided at that time. In November, Basil was hospitalized because his intense pain caused him to vomit so much that he was becoming dehydrated. At one point, we didn't think he was going to pull through. Somehow, he stabilized, and we were able to bring him home. That night and the next morning he got worse again; this time it was bad enough that I thought we were going to lose him. I called Deb and told her that if they were going to graduate Bubby, they had better do it now. That morning Deb called the superintendent who agreed to contact all members of the school board to get a diploma signed and ready for Basil. They worked quickly, and on that day, November 6, 1990, the Bluffton-

Harrison School Board and Superintendent Gary McMillen awarded Basil his high school diploma. Present at the ceremony at our home were Basil Sr. and me, Superintendent McMillen, school board members Kenneth Ellenberger and Ann Flanningham, Assistant Superintendent Thomas Byanski, Bluffton High School Principal Frank O'Shea, Wells County Assessor Connie Prible (sister of Deb Johnson), Special Services Director Jackie Wolpert, and Deb Johnson, Basil's special teacher. I so appreciate the willingness of the school corporation to make one of Basil's primary goals come true.

Soon after receiving his diploma Basil entered the hospital, again vomiting and dehydrating due to the severe head pain. Dr. Fischer started a morphine drip through his IV. Even though for the last few months Basil had been in the hospital different times, this was one time I will always remember. My husband's brothers expressed concern that I had agreed for Bubby to be put on the morphine drip. When I found this out, I let it upset me so much that I became sick myself. I guess I just couldn't handle any differing opinions then, even those with good intentions. All I knew was that my son needed me there with all the love and support that I could possibly give him. I simply could not allow myself to get sick, physically or emotionally. While my sister sat in the room with Basil, I took a walk by myself to think things out. I found myself remembering all the times Basil had been sick in his seventeen years of life. I thought about who was always there and knew how he suffered with broken bones over the years, and who was there now holding his ribs, praying he wouldn't break them or maybe even puncture a lung while vomiting or coughing with a cold or pneumonia. I was that person, and that's how it should be. I was his mother, and nobody knew his needs or loved him as I did. So I went back into my son's room, knowing I had made the right decision about the morphine drip. I felt we had a sensitive, intelligent doctor, and we had a lot of faith in her judgement.

I knew in my heart the family was only thinking of Basil's well-being. But I really believe that unless you are the one giving care to a desperately ill person and are with that person constantly, you cannot understand how the parents suffer. Our doctor even said that she often would like to remove a patient from all pain medication so that other family members could see how the patient suffered; but she, of course, would never do that to a patient. She did understand how quick people are to judge others when we really don't know what they are going through. The fact is that as parents, we shed many tears over our children and we try to do everything possible to keep them from suffering, and I was no different than any other mother.

I do thank my mother-in-law for her kind words to me before leaving the hospital to go home. She said, "Dorothy, you've been a wonderful mother to Basil in giving him all the love and care possible over the years. Anything you feel should be done for our grandson, we are with you all the way because you know his needs better than anyone." At that time, her words and support meant more to me that I can ever express.

During Basil's stay in the hospital this time, his respirations were extremely low. One day a nurse named Ronnie came into the room and stood beside Basil's bed. He had been so bad that I guess the nurse felt she had to be realistic with us. She told my husband and me (along with my sister, sister-in-law, and Deb) that we needed to prepare ourselves because Basil Jr. wasn't going to live. We sobbed and sobbed, trying to console each other. To this day, I believe that Basil Jr. heard what Ronnie had said and knew how upset his dad and I were. I think his sheer determination to hold on overpowered his fragile body. Basil soon snapped back after that, and before long we were bringing him home again.

Basil Grows Up

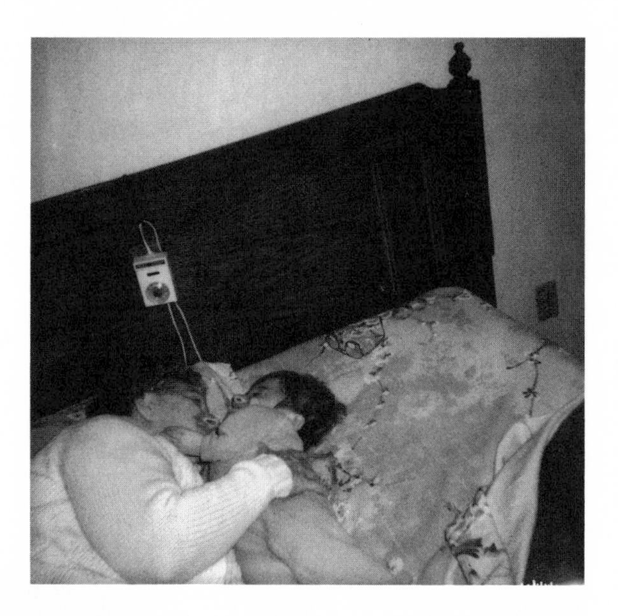

Grandma Sarah, here shown at her house, was a favorite.

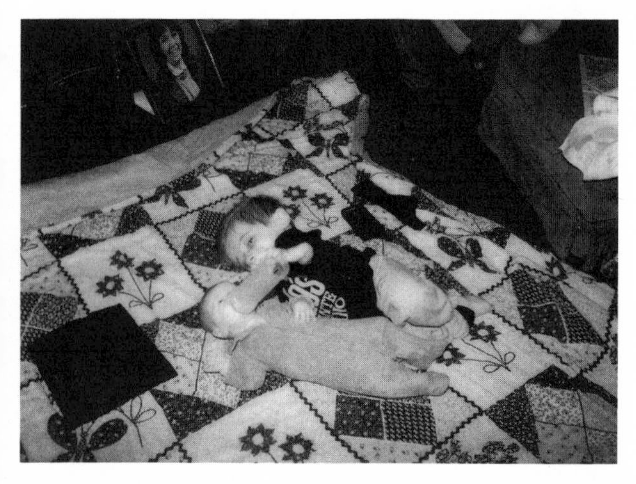

At eleven, Basil enjoyed feeding his cousin, J.C.

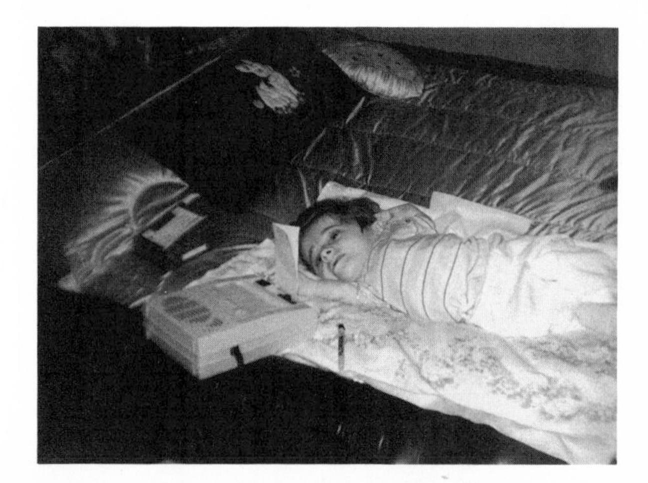

Cassettes were an important part of class.

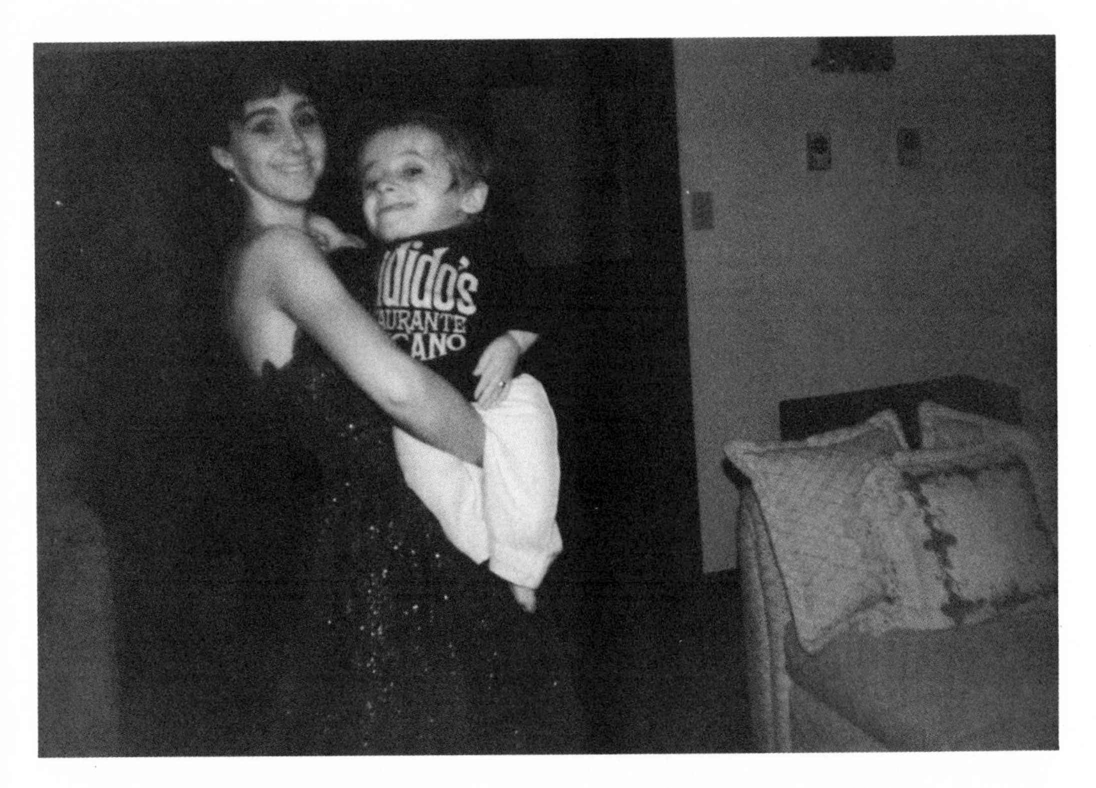

Priscilla goes to the Jr.-Sr. Prom. Basil wishes her well.(l)

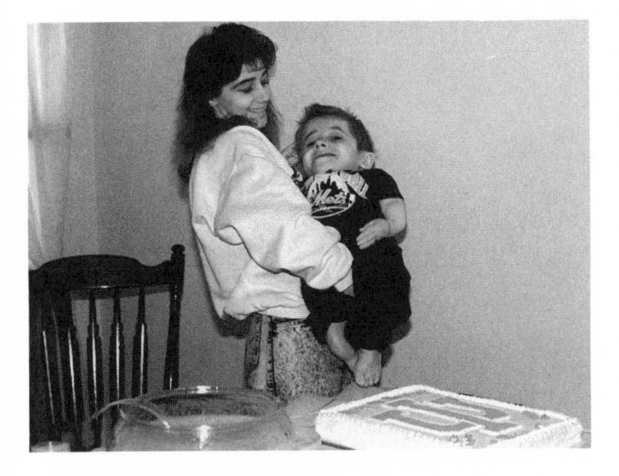

Priscilla helped Basil enjoy
an IU cake at his 16th
birthday party.

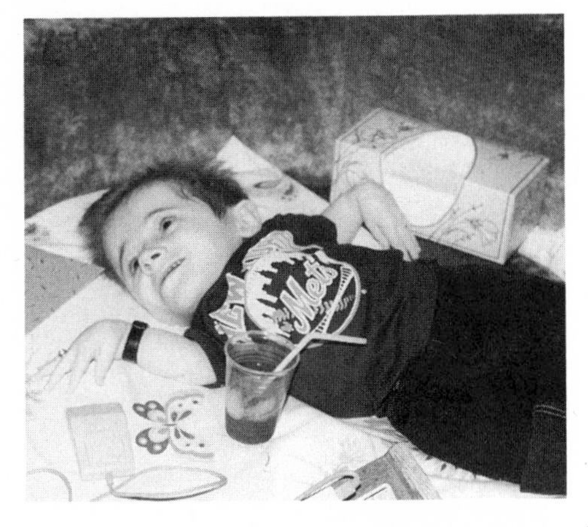

Basil looked at cards
and talked with friends
at the party. Note the
ever-present iced tea.

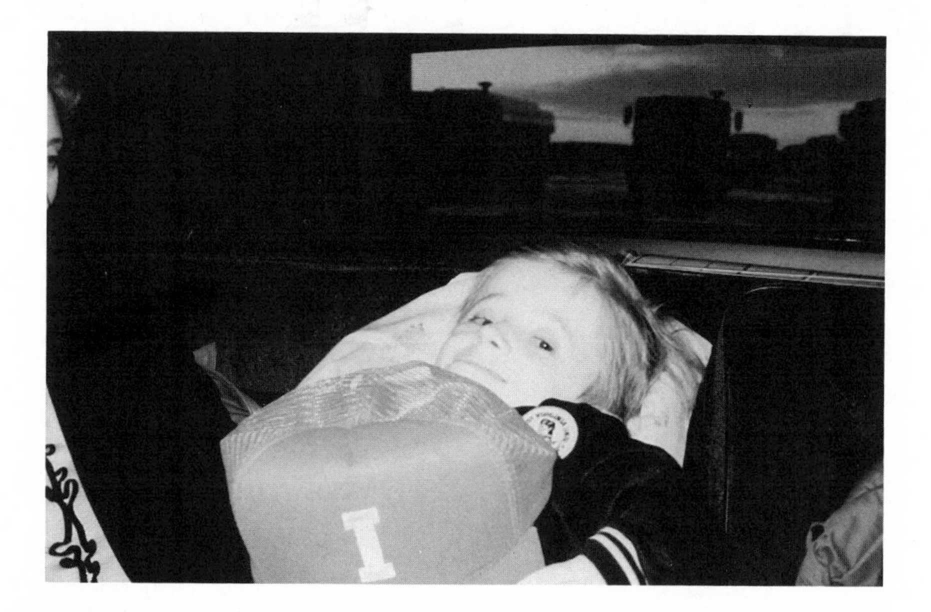

At Baer Field Airport, Basil met Indiana basketball players just before a scrimmage.

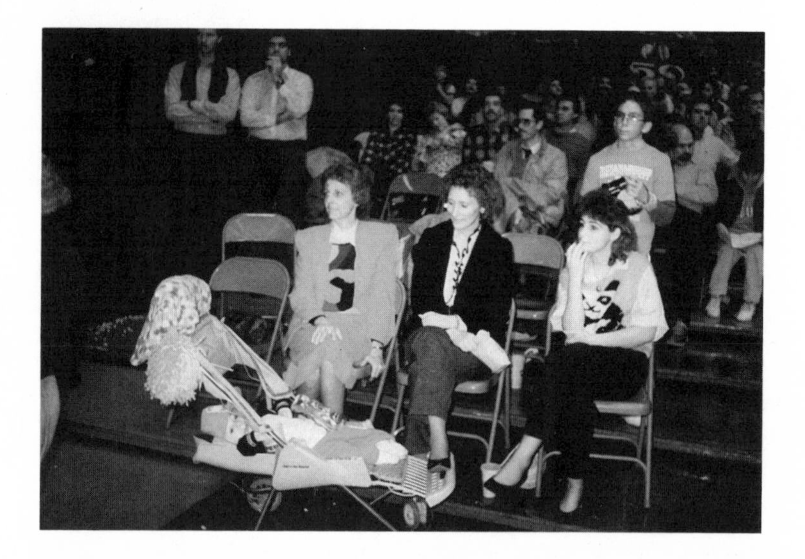

In Fort Wayne, Basil, with his mother, sister, and 6th grade teacher, Sally Shively, watched his favorite team, IU, play a game.

THE LAST FEW YEARS OF BASIL'S LIFE

Even though Basil's school days were over and his pain unbearable, I tried to keep him as active as possible. Trying to find interesting activities for my intelligent and "with-it" son was nothing new—Basil always enjoyed life to the fullest.

Before he grew very ill, there were trips to take. His favorite place to visit was in Akron, Ohio, at his Aunt Nora's and Uncle John's home. His Aunt Nora always planned a full schedule for him while he was there. We always left it up to him if he was feeling well enough to go out for the day. Very seldom did he refuse.

Because of Basil's physical handicap, I felt it was more important than usual for him to see and do all he possibly could for himself. Mentally, Basil was a very intelligent young man who was trapped in the body of an infant. But he never complained. I always told him God gave him a good mind to use, and in many ways that could prove to be more useful to him than a strong and healthy body ever could.

One vacation that especially stands out in my mind was when we took Basil to Canada and rented a cottage at the lake for a week. He wanted to fish off the dock, but because Basil had such delicate skin, I had to be careful about having him in the sun for long periods of time. Basil's cousin David came up with the idea of making a tent for him. All we had were two chairs and a blanket. I laid Bubby between the chairs in his seat, and we stretched the blanket over the chairs like a tent. David and Basil fished for a couple of hours that afternoon. I'm not sure who wiggled the most—Basil or the fish he caught! The next day Basil wanted to go out on the lake in a row boat, so later in the evening we took him. I remember him saying, "Mom, the sunset sure is beautiful, and it's so quiet and peaceful way out here on the lake." I guess our desire to give him a great vacation overshadowed any fear we may have had about the boat tipping. We really didn't think about all of the possible risks; we just took him. If we worried about every possible danger to our son, he would not have had any kind of life at all. He just would have been in bed his whole life; even though one doctor actually suggested something like that, we could not ever have done that to our child.

Basil said that his most memorable time in Canada was riding in a glider. I had a terrible fear of letting him go in the glider, especially during takeoff and landing. The water was rough, and I dreaded the thought of Basil suffering yet another broken bone during his fun vacation. But I knew how important this ride was to him. The ride was a little rough while on the water, but once we got in the air Basil really enjoyed himself. The pilot gave him a set of headphones to put on so he could tell him about all the different islands in that area. But to be honest, I believe Basil talked more than the pilot! He probably asked more questions in those thirty minutes than the pilot usually had in a day's time. I recall as I stepped off the glider with Basil in my arms how he looked at me and said, "That sure was a lot of fun, Mom!" That made all my anxiety worth it.

Basil loved sports. He enjoyed and collected baseball cards. His highlight was buying, selling and trading with the card dealers. Let me tell you, Basil never came out on the short end of any deal! His shrewd little mind always made sure that he profited in some way from the deals. Nobody could take advantage of him, even if they wanted to. We would roll him into the card shop in his stroller. Once the owner got over the shock of an adult voice coming out of this little body, he would start talking "shop" with Basil. They all realized that Basil knew what he was talking about. I think they all enjoyed doing business with him. There was only one bad experience. One time Basil, Jeremy, and Brady went card shopping together. Basil bought an entire box of cards; it was supposed to have been an entire set. When we got home, the boys opened the box and began sorting through all of those cards. Suddenly, Basil realized that three of the most valuable cards were missing. He said, "Mom, we've been cheated!" Of course, I had to take the box back to the dealer on my way to work that day. I talked to Basil that evening from work and told him the dealer apologized and said that he sometimes had school kids make up the boxes; it had just been a mistake. When Basil heard that, he said, "Right. It's a funny thing that they just happened to leave out the good cards." He didn't miss a trick with his cards. Actually, he really didn't even trust me to do his trading! He would let me buy for him, because we could write down exactly what he wanted. But when it came to trading, if he couldn't go himself, I had to take Jeremy or Brady along because they "knew what they were doing."Another sport he really enjoyed was basketball, especially college basketball. His all-time favorite team was the Indiana University Hoosiers, coached by Bob Knight. He loved watching the televised games, talking about them, listening to games on the radio, and collecting souvenirs of all kinds. He even had a headband that said "Indiana University" and he couldn't even wear headbands! Coach Bob Knight was generous—he kept in touch with Basil. He even called us on the phone a couple of times so he could talk with Basil. He also sent an autographed basketball for Basil's sixteenth birthday party given by Deb and Evelyn in March 1990. Basil received a card from Coach Knight during one of his longer stays in the hospital. Regardless of what people think of Coach Knight, I know he has a big heart. When the Hoosiers played their scrimmage in Fort Wayne, Indiana, we took Basil to the airport to meet the team when they arrived. Basil got to shake hands with Coach Knight and all of the players. It was a cold day, so we kept Basil in the car. They all stopped by the car and reached through the window to shake hands and say a few words. Not all well-known people care to take the time for someone special like Basil. He liked following the better IU players when they would go pro. One of his favorites was Isiah Thomas, who went on to play with the Detroit Pistons. Isiah took the time to send autographed pictures to our son. Basil almost worshipped these guys. We still have all of the autographed books, balls, and other IU mementos that Basil collected. He enjoyed showing them off, and I guess we just don't want to give them up.

Although basketball was Basil's favorite sport, he also liked pro football and baseball. His football team was the Dallas Cowboys; he always rooted for them during football season. When it came to football teams, it didn't matter how many wins or losses, Basil was still for the Cowboys all the way. His favorite baseball team was the New York Mets; he also followed the Cincinnati Reds, probably because they were Jeremy's and Brady's team. Even when the Mets had losing seasons, Basil still cheered them on. He especially liked the players Dwight Gooden and Darryl Strawberry. Basil tried to be supportive of them even when they had severe personal problems that made the national news. When the Make-a-Wish Foundation contacted Basil about his wish, he finally decided that he would like to meet Gooden and Strawberry. The Foundation was attempting to set up a meeting sometime when the Mets would play near our home. They were hoping the two players would be able to stop by our motel on the way to the game. However, they had to call back with the disappointing news that the comment had been made, "It just upsets me too much to be around sick kids." There was no way I was going to tell Basil that; for the first and last time, I lied to him. I made up a story about us not being able to find a motel with a suitable water bed for him. I knew that it would have broken his heart to know the truth. One of those players did end up calling Basil on the phone and talking for a couple of minutes. The way I look at it now is that it was their loss, not Basil's.

Because of his enthusiasm for sports, Basil became quite a little celebrity among the local sports media in our area. A Fort Wayne radio station, WOWO, hosted a radio talk show called "Sportstalk." Listeners could phone in during this live broadcast and offer comments or ask questions about any sport. The co-hosts were Dean Pantazi and Art Saltsberg who worked in radio and television sports broadcasting. Of course, Basil liked calling in to talk with Dean and Art. He called so often that he became friends with the cohosts. Some nights when Basil did not call, Dean and Art would even mention Basil on the air. They knew of his loyalty to the Mets and IU basketball, and they teased him constantly about being a Mets fan because New York is so far away from Indiana; most Hoosiers are fans of either the Cubs or the Reds. Basil took it well, especially when the Mets had a good season. He loved to rub it in! Art was good about supporting Basil whenever he could; he attended the ceremony when Basil was presented with the Young Heroes' Medal of Honor.

Attractions

And

Diversions

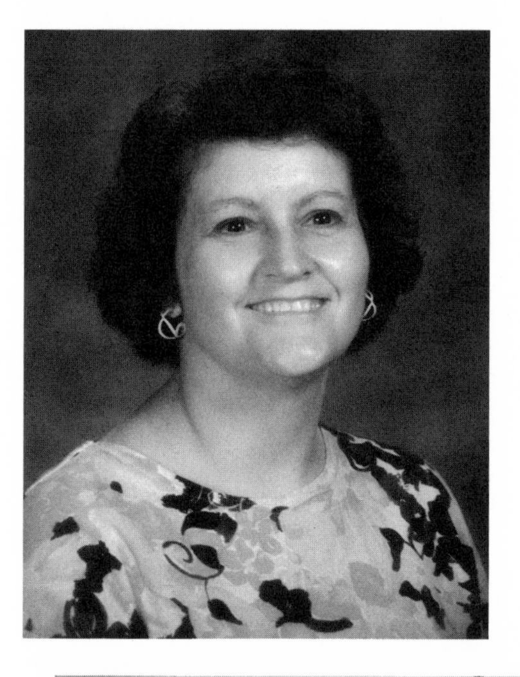

Basil loved, and gave his best work to high school teacher Deb Johnson.

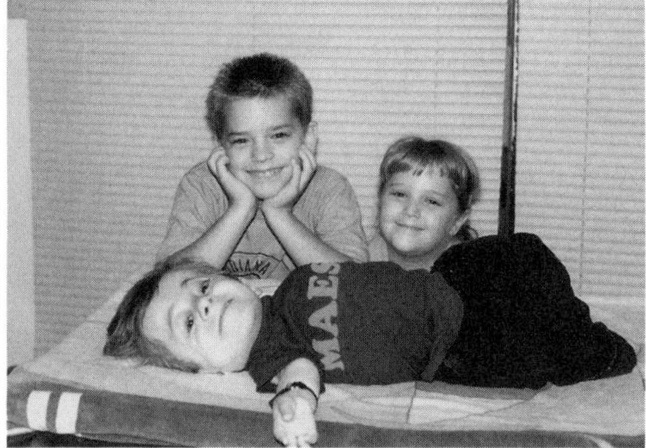

Basil enjoyed being with Adam and Lori Beth Johnson, Deb's children.

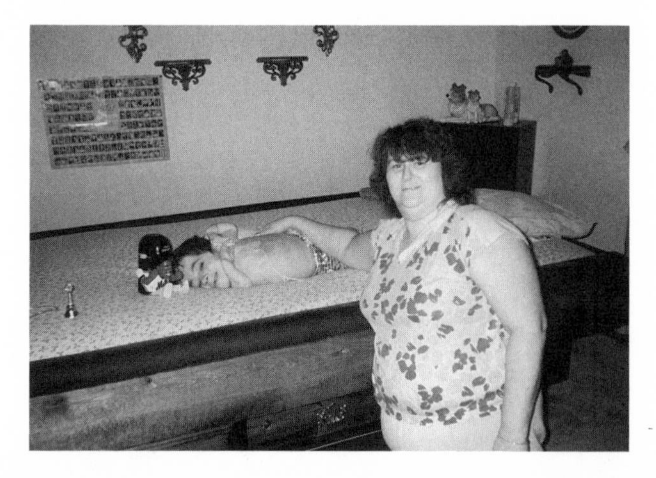

Aunt Nora Casto played a special role always in Basil's life.

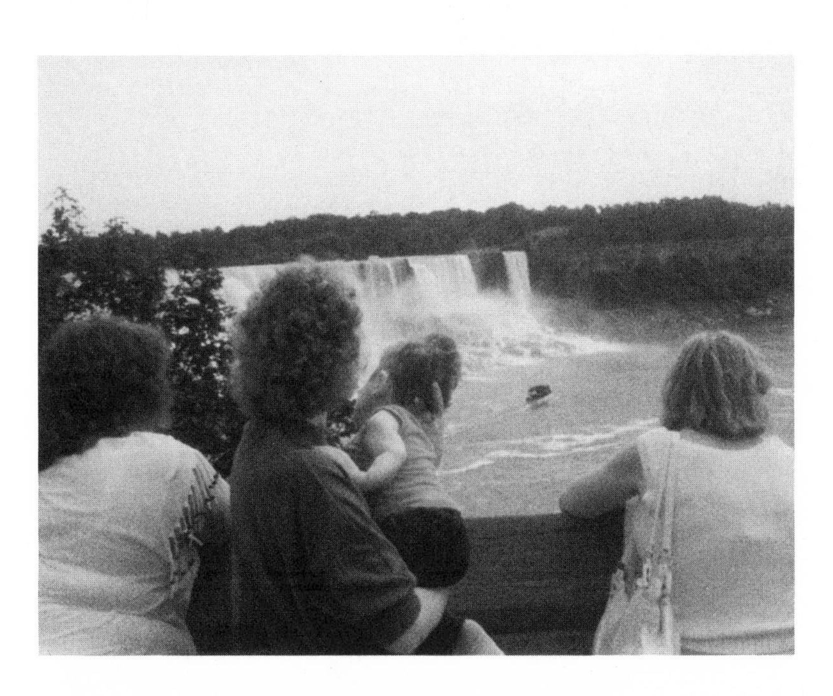

Niagara Falls was fascinating to Basil, his mother and Aunt Nora.

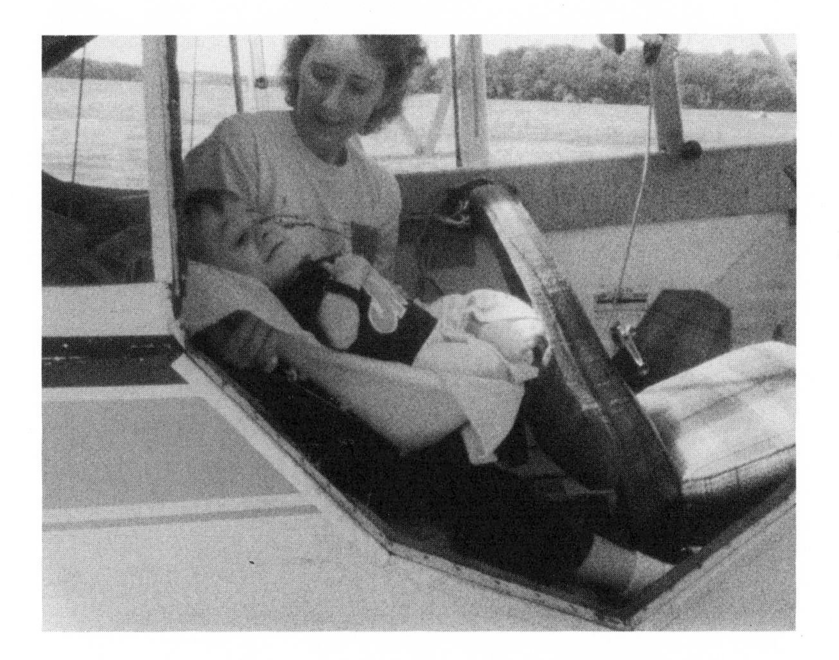

Basil and his apprehensive mother sat in a glider ready to check out the islands around the lake in Canada.

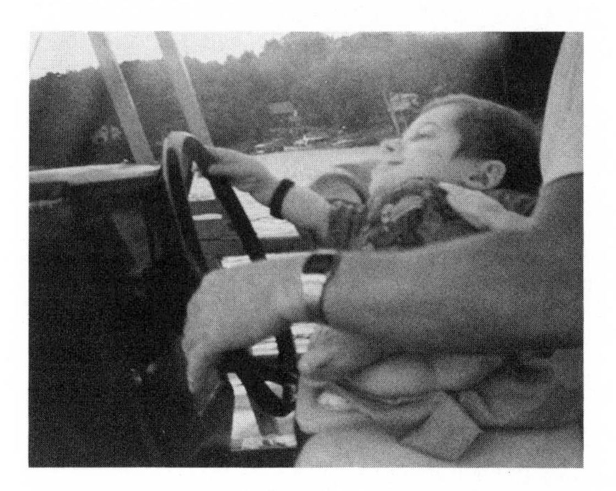

A ride in his Uncle John's boat gave our hero a chance to steer.

Basil, here with Uncle John,visited the Football Hall of Fame.

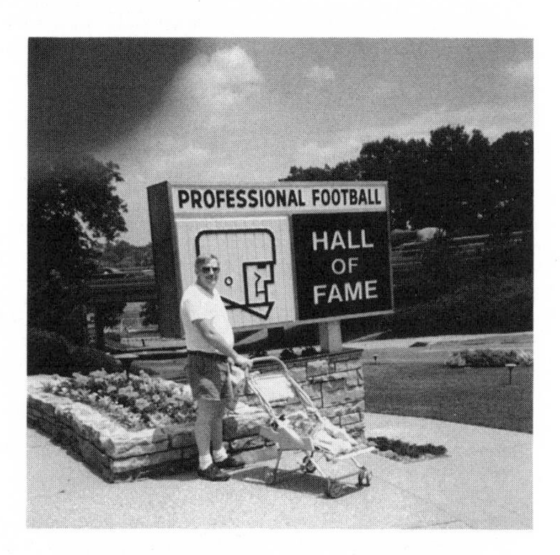

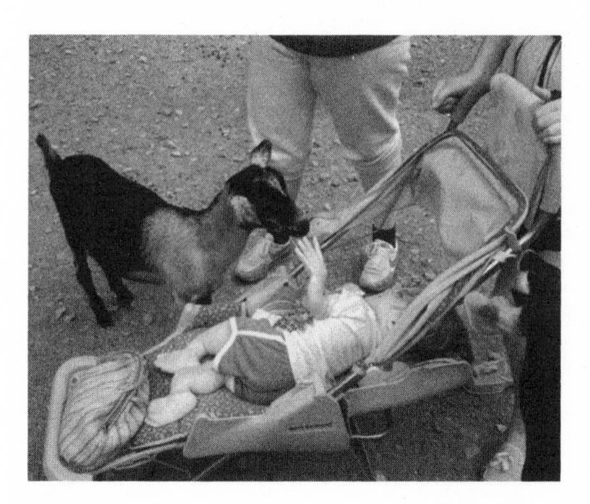

Goats were one of the animals Basil enjoyed while visiting the Akron Zoo.

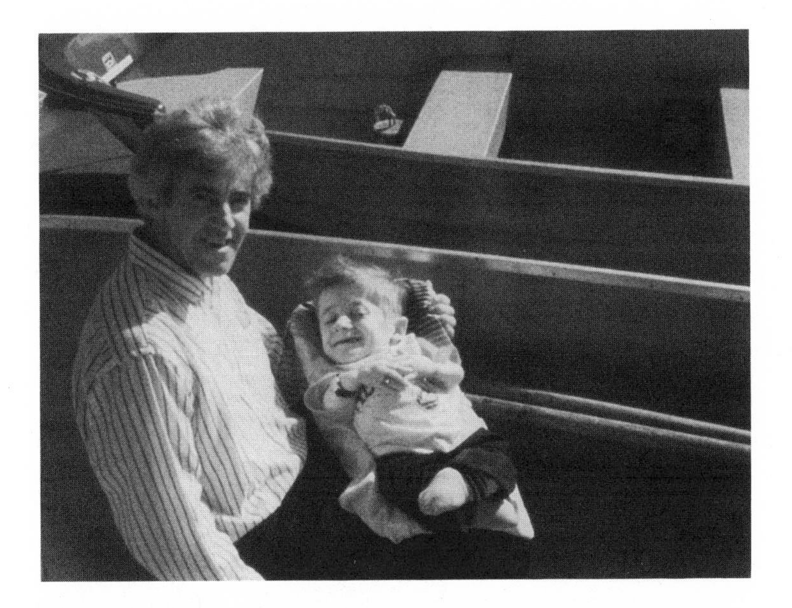

Basil in Canada was ready for a ride on the lake with his Dad.

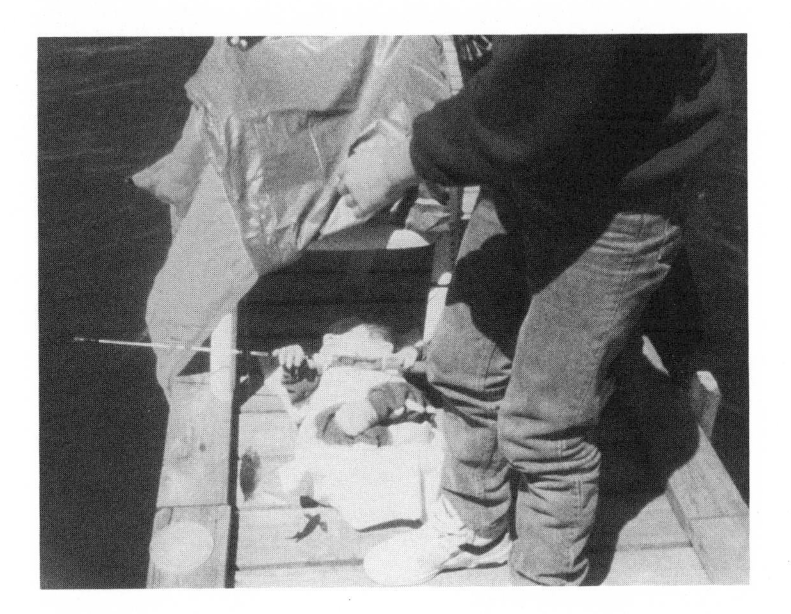

Fishing off the dock with cousin David, while vacationing in Canada was a lot of fun.

A real highlight for all of us was in the summer of '91 when Dean and Art were able to come to our home to do a live broadcast for Sportstalk. This was made possible through the Make-a-Wish Foundation since the other wish (to meet Gooden and Strawberry) could not be arranged. They arrived loaded with microphones, sports stats, and the station's mobile unit. Basil was so excited, and even a little nervous. His big moment finally arrived, and he even had his own mike! Dean and Art allowed Basil to answer some of the questions that were phoned in. The three of them had a great time together, and the hour passed all too quickly for Basil. As the program neared its end, Basil quietly whispered to Dean, "May I do the closing?" Dean said he could. Basil's debut as a radio co-host ended with the words, "This is WOWO. For Art and Dean, this is Basil. Good night."

One of our local newspaper editors, Joe Smekens, became friends with our Basil, too, and became Basil's reporter, detailing his activities in the newspaper. He knew Basil's love for sports, and was always looking for ways to involve Basil in the great Hoosier sport. A new museum was built in New Castle, Indiana, to honor high school basketball. For a time, residents could "buy" a brick with their name on it that would be used in making a walkway into the museum. Joe was kind enough to get a brick for Basil; even though Basil was never able to see it, there is a brick with his name on it at the Indiana High School Basketball Hall of Fame in New Castle, Indiana.

Basil thought that was wonderful. Deb Johnson and her family visited the museum a few years ago and told me about seeing the brick. Joe and his brother, Mike, had become pretty close to Basil because Mike had a son with a similar condition. Mike's son, Scott, lived in Florida with his mother, so Mike and Joe didn't get to see him as often as they would have liked. It helped them to be with Basil, and it helped Basil because he liked them so well. Even today, we keep in touch with Joe and Mike.

Another of Basil's special pleasures was shopping. He could almost outshop his mother! Because he had to be having a really good day for us to go, trips to the shopping mall were infrequent. He loved buying new clothes, like most teenagers. Jewelry was another favorite, especially anything gold. We even had a class ring made for him; it had to be special ordered because his finger was so small. And, of course, he really liked the expensive stuff the most! We did buy him a gold chain and a gold ring with a tiny diamond in it, and he enjoyed wearing those whenever he dressed up for church or pictures. He always made a point to hold his hand so that his ring would show in a picture. I have to admit clothing was sometimes difficult to find. Basil knew what he wanted, but it was hard for us to find things that didn't look too childish. Usually I'd have to hem the pants and cut off the sleeves to make them fit. One thing that helped is when the fashions changed so that even adults were wearing Mickey Mouse and other cartoon characters on clothing. Those clothes we could find in his size. Basil's shopping included checking out the latest Nintendo games and Christian rock tapes. The clerks at some of the stores got to know us pretty well. Most of them were kind and eager to help Basil in his decisions. And that wasn't always easy! Part of our fun was eating at the mall before we returned home.

One of Basil's favorite rock groups was Stryper. He always checked to see if they had any new CD's out when we went shopping. He owned his own CD player which he received from his fellow high school students through a fund raiser called "Buckets for Santa." The PE teacher, Tony Garton, sponsors this worthy endeavor every year to raise money for some worthwhile project. Basil ended up buying all the Stryper CD's he could find.

Stryper, which had started out as a Christian rock group, but had also decided to do secular music, went on tour. Basil thought it would be wonderful to go to a Stryper concert. When I heard that they would be in Fort Wayne in January 1992, I knew I had to take Basil.

The weather was awful the day of the concert. The roads were snowy and icy; but we plodded ahead anyway. We had four tickets, so we took two of our friends along. Jeremy and Brady could not go, so Basil was stuck with three women! We made it safely, and everyone was so considerate of Basil and his illness. The pastor of the Vineyard Christian Fellowship met us at the door and unlocked the nursery so we could wait there until Stryper arrived. Within a few minutes, Stryper arrived. Basil had pictures taken with them before and after the concert. They guys introduced themselves and talked with Basil awhile. They all wore little sunglasses, so they let Basil try on a pair. All of them were so kind to Bubby. They put us right on stage, near a speaker. A young man was assigned to us to protect Basil from the crowd. This was a rock concert, so you can imagine the volume of sound on that stage! Basil didn't mind the noise because he was having such a great time. He even sang along with them. After the concert, we went to the van to start home. Then Basil admitted that his head hurt terribly and he thought he was going to vomit. But it had been worth it to Basil to have had such a memorable evening.

Friends were very important to Basil. He often wished his classmates would come out for visits, but it didn't happen very often. I explained that it was hard for other kids to take the time to drive six miles south of town to visit him when they all were busy with school, jobs, and dating. He understood, but it still hurt his feelings. One classmate, though, was very good about coming to visit. Chris Mettler called Basil a lot on the phone, and they got to know each other better that way. Once Chris got his license, he drove out to visit Bubby quite a bit. They talked baseball cards and music. Chris played the guitar, so he would give us a little concert every now and then. He often brought his girlfriend, Cami Reber, with him. Cami was so good to Basil, too; they both brought out Christmas gifts for him. Chris wanted Basil to go to their junior prom at the high school so badly, but Basil just wasn't well enough to go. Chris still came out on prom night to show Basil his tux. We took pictures with Bubby holding Chris's walking stick. I'll always appreciate those two teenagers who took the extra time and effort to include Basil in their lives.

Yes, Basil missed his prom, and a good deal more by this time. His illness was getting bad enough that we no longer lived our normal lifestyle. His pain had intensified enough that his regular pain medicine simply was not working. The doctors tried some stronger pain relievers. One medication was effective for the pain, but it tore up his stomach so much that he couldn't eat. He was also vomiting more, so that aggravated his stomach even more. We had to find another medication that would work to give him some time free from the torment his condition was now bringing. Dr. Fischer decided to try Roxanol, a fast-acting form of morphine that is held under the tongue and absorbed. This seemed to be effective, but the problem was it had to be given every hour around the clock. Basil had to stay awake long enough for the Roxanol to be absorbed; this meant that he (actually all of us) couldn't ever sleep more than forty-five minutes at a time. Once his body got used to the medicine, we had to increase the dosage in order for it to be effective. This means it took longer for his body to absorb it, which means even less sleep per hour. I can honestly say this was a horrible time for all of us. Basil was at a very challenging point in his life. I had nurses in my home to help, but on quite a few occasions Basil had no nurse. If my sister-in-law, Janet, had not helped me, I'd never have survived all the hours of staying awake to make sure my son had his pain medicine. Janet wasn't comfortable drawing Basil's Roxanol into the syringes, so I'd always get eight hours of medicine ready and lay the syringes on a paper towel with the time each should be given written above it. This way there was no confusion between Janet and me as to when the last dose had been administered. Basil was on Roxanol for approximately six weeks. I started noticing the dark circles under Bubby's eyes. What really hurt was that he had no joy in life anymore. Life became a struggle to just endure one hour to the next. By then I knew he couldn't go on the rest of his life never getting a full hour of sleep at a time, let alone a whole night of rest. Janet and I each had an alarm clock set, the timer on my cook stove was set, and my husband also bought me a clock that chimed every hour. Still we worried about missing his medication. It was a very difficult time in our lives; most people cannot understand the worry or fatigue we all suffered. As it was, my son could never have had any pleasure out of life at all, and as we've shown, Basil was a young man who wanted to live life to the fullest. That's when I knew that something had to change. In talking with Dr. Fischer, I realized that our last hope was a central line to get the morphine directly into his bloodstream.

Dr. Fischer discussed the potential dangers of putting in a central line. First, Basil could not be anesthetized because his respiratory system could not tolerate it. Putting in a central line is a surgical procedure, so he would have to endure it with just a local anesthetic. She also told us that once the line was put in, and he was on a morphine drip, he had to keep the line. There was no turning back. We felt like we really had no alternative but to go with the central line. Fortunately, Dr. Fischer could recommend a good surgeon at Riley Children's Hospital in Indianapolis. She said that it was going to be a tricky procedure, but if anybody could put a central line in Bubby, Dr. Fred Rescorla could.

On February 27, 1991, Dr. Rescorla put a central line in Basil so he could get his morphine continuously with a PCA pump at home. Basil had such severe pain, and the central line eliminated the need for inserting a regular IV so frequently. Going into the operating room with strangers and knowing how dangerous the surgery was made this one of the most frightening times of his life. Basil said, "Mom, it was scary in that big room with all the doctors standing over me, but the worst thing about it all was you not being there to handle me." Basil's collar bone was broken due to the pressure put on it when the line was put in; the doctors had expected that and had explained it to us before surgery. We survived the surgery, but we were warned that his line had to be kept open. If it clogged, we would have to take him back to Indianapolis and have a new line put in. The thought of Basil facing surgery again was frightening. We knew it was imperative that we keep an eye on the central line to make sure it stayed open. The real problem was that morphine is addictive; we knew our son would be addicted to the drug. If the line clogged up, he would not get the morphine and he would be thrown into withdrawal. That could cause him severe problems because of the vomiting and extreme body convulsions associated with withdrawal. Basil could easily break his neck or back under those conditions. Plus, his pain would have been intolerable. So it became my number one priority to keep checking that line.

At home I had to keep nurses to help out so I could rest at night. Their primary responsibility was to make certain that line stayed open. The morphine was in a small cassette that fit into a PCA pump, which was designed to beep if the drug ran out, if the line clogged, or if the line was clamped off. This was portable enough so that we could travel with it. I had some problems with a few nurses who wanted to sleep during their midnight shifts. One night I got up to use the bathroom and I heard this snoring. I went out to check, and Basil's nurse was so sound asleep that he was snoring. I knew that at 5:00 Basil needed some antibiotic added to his line; I decided to wait and see if the nurse would wake up. He had his watch alarm set, and he did wake up for the 5:00 medicine. I confronted him about being asleep, and he said he was only dozing. I told him I had been sitting there for a half hour listening to his snoring and I knew he was not just dozing. I told him to get his shoes on, go home, and not come back. When Bubby found out that I fired this nurse, he cried and cried because that was his favorite nurse. This may seem a bit harsh, but I had to keep Basil's welfare as my top concern. I had to fire two other nurses for sleeping on that night shift. I simply couldn't rest if I had to worry about that line clogging up while the nurse was sleeping. Home nurses can be a wonderful help when things are done as they should be done and we did have some very responsible nurses, too. The ones I fired were actually very good nurses; I guess they just slacked off in their duties after they had been here awhile.

Before we ever left Riley, the nurses told me that I had to learn to change the dressing on Basil's central line. Even though they knew I would have nursing help, it was absolutely essential that one person take care of the line all the time. The hospital nurses suggested that I be the one to do it. Everything had to be kept sterile because any infection would cause the line to have to be removed. It had been a big risk putting the first one in, and the doctor had stated it was necessary that this line be kept in. He was surprised that Basil had survived the first surgery, and he felt certain that he would not survive a second one. After they showed me how to do it, I had to practice with a special pillow. Once I felt I knew what I was doing, I had to do the procedure in front of the nurses. They then assured me that we were ready to go home.

Dr. Fischer helped us in so many ways. I will always be indebted to her. She really had to do some talking with our insurance company to convince them that Basil should be able to stay at home. Once they understood Dr. Fischer's viewpoint, they agreed to help cover the expenses of keeping Basil at home. And we had expenses! His morphine cassettes cost about $250 each; he went through two a day. The nursing was expensive, too. In the beginning, I only had a nurse for an eight hour night shift; later, I had a nurse for sixteen hours. Toward the end, I had a nurse here about eighteen hours a day, unless the agency had trouble getting enough help.

Dr. Fischer also willingly came to the house to check on Basil instead of demanding we take him to town to her office. Sometimes Dr. Dian would come out in the mornings before going to his office so he could check Basil. I always fixed him a big breakfast and he would eat as we discussed Basil's health problems. I hope he enjoyed the breakfasts as much as I appreciated his coming out to visit Basil at home.

Since the PCA pump was portable, we were able to travel. And, of course, Basil wanted to go see Aunt Nora. On one of our visits with Nora, we took Basil to the Pro Football Hall of Fame. He was so excited! His big brown eyes sparkled, especially when we came to the players' diamond rings on display. Another time we decided to take him out for a ride in my sister's speed boat. That was a challenge! We put Basil in a portable crib and tied it inside the boat. This way he could see. Then we held an umbrella over him to protect him from the sun. When Uncle John started the engine, Bubby said, "Put the pedal to the metal, Uncle John!" Well, I'm glad John didn't. Shortly after starting the boat, a water patrol officer stopped us to see what was going on. Nora was certain we would get a ticket, but all he said was to drive slowly and carefully, and have a good time with Basil! Another time we took Bubby to Sea World in Aurora, Ohio. He loved to watch the killer whales. Basil had his picture taken with the Shamu characters. He was having a pretty good day, so he was able to enjoy his visit at Sea World. We bought him a short set and a Shamu piggy bank. He wanted to go back for a second visit later on, but it never worked out. We had reservations for a nice motel because Basil wanted to stay in "a really nice place," two rooms because John and Nora went with us. It was costing us more than we normally would have spent, but it was all for Bubby. As soon as we arrived, we put him on the bed. He grinned and said, "Room service, please!" He had a dish of chocolate ice cream while Uncle John enjoyed some coffee. Later that evening, Basil became really sick. We had to start an IV solution for him; our nurse was with us, so she did it. We had to call our doctor back home for instructions. We ended up spending the night, but the next morning we headed back to Nora's. So Basil never made it back to Sea World again. We finished our visit with Nora and John, and then returned home as we had planned.

The rest of that summer and fall brought no improvement in Basil's health; he didn't get a lot worse, but he sure didn't get any better. He still had his severe headaches, along with the vomiting. We had to increase the morphine every few days to help him tolerate the pain. His appetite was still normal, and I was thankful for that. I was also thankful for the friends who continued to stop in to visit Bubby. Jeremy and Brady still played Nintendo. They used their nicknames for each other: Basil was "Big Guy," Jeremy was "Small Fry," and Brady was "The Bradster." Basil told them he felt as if they were all brothers. Even after Basil became so ill, the boys were available and ready to be friends. If Bubby asked for something to drink, or even an ice pack for his head, one of them always jumped up and got it for him.

Basil always loved company. James and Cheryl, our good friends of many years, came to visit him often. They went through baseball cards with him; he enjoyed discussing certain players with James. Believe me, they never agreed on much of anything! James and Basil simply enjoyed teasing each other. Ron and Kathy, more of our friends, visited often, too. Whenever they came, we all knew the discussion was going to be IU basketball. Both Basil and Kathy were big IU fans, and they loved Bobby Knight as a coach.

During the summer of 1991, we had a prowler in our neighborhood. We were concerned, of course, but especially concerned because of the large amount of morphine we had to keep on hand in our home. A lot of people knew about Basil's being on morphine, so we always worried about the possibility of a break-in. The sheriff's department was called and the gentleman on duty was Deputy Mike Smekens. I had known of Mike, of course, but this was the first time he had been to our house. While he was at our house, he came in for a minute to meet Basil. As Mike was leaving, Basil told him to stop in anytime. Mike said, "I sure will." From that evening on, Basil and Mike were best friends. When Mike could, he'd stop in to watch a ball game, play a little golf on the Nintendo, or do anything to keep Basil company. They even painted a picture together and called it "Bobby Knight's Hideaway" because the cabin had a bright red roof (IU color). Mike's wife, Melissa, and his children Chad and Amy also came out to visit with Basil. Mike even brought his parents out to meet Basil. Joe, Mike's brother, came out to watch a ball game with them one evening. Basil enjoyed that a lot. I wish I had the words to tell Mike how much Basil loved and admired him.

When Christmas or Basil's birthday came around, he received cards from classmates, friends, family, and a lot of wonderful people in our community. During the time Basil was extremely ill, he received cards from many people just to let him know they were praying for him and thinking of him often. Those prayers, I know, helped us all.

Basil was a strong believer in God and enjoyed reading and learning all he possibly could from his Bible. He was disappointed that he couldn't hold a Bible and read it himself. For Christmas one year, Deb gave him the Bible on cassettes. He enjoyed listening to the dramatic readings of the Scriptures. Basil became an adult member of the Park United Brethren Church on August 20, 1991. Usually on Saturday evenings he would say to me, "Mom, if I'm able, I'd like to go to church in the morning." After Basil became so ill, he only made it to church a couple of Sunday mornings. Even so, that never discouraged Basil from his faith and love for God. Pastor Dave came to visit Basil frequently. They both enjoyed talking about sports for awhile, and then Pastor Dave would read to Basil from the Bible and have prayer with him. I remember distinctly one Tuesday afternoon when Pastor Dave left that Basil commented to me that he felt no one truly realized how much pain he was in but God. Maybe that was why Basil felt so close to Him at all times.

Basil discussed his feelings about everything with me and I'm sure that's the reason we had such a binding love and closeness with each other. Evidently it stood out to everyone immediately after seeing us together. Basil had a nurse named Melba who had been to our home a few times. Melba was a very wise and caring nurse. She realized Basil was in extreme pain; not only his head, but his entire body hurt. I recall the night Melba came into my kitchen and said, "Dorothy, I hope you don't think I'm out of line, but I see the closeness between Basil and you which I admire very much. But you need to realize the only reason Basil is fighting so hard to live is because of you." Melba didn't tell me a thing that I hadn't already said to myself. I knew she was right; I had to be the one to tell my son he was not going to get better this time. But how do you tell a son that awful truth? When do you tell him?

Basil wanted to go home with his Aunt Nora around the middle of March when she came up for a visit, so we did. I was hesitant to go; Basil was sick and vomiting when we left, but he said, "Mom, I can be sick in Ohio the same as at home." Before we left I started an IV on Bubby for the vomiting. This was through his central line, and he was feeling somewhat better. Dr. Fischer had said earlier in the week that a trip would be good for him, especially a trip to Aunt Nora's. Even though Basil left with an IV running and we had to stop along the way to put a catheter in for him, I'm very thankful we went. Now that I think about it, I believe Bubby knew his time on earth was getting much shorter.

While in Ohio, Basil became comatose. We were terrified, but we knew that such high dosages of morphine could cause such a reaction. Nora and I took him to see Dr. Wiener, whom Basil had seen before. Because of Basil's severe head pain, he referred Basil to a neurologist named Dr. Timmons. Dr. Timmons looked into Basil's eyes and said to me, "You have no idea how sick your son is, or the severity of his pain." While at the hospital, Basil had a CAT scan done, along with some blood work. Dr. Timmons said he could see something behind Basil's left eye, but a good view of the left side of his head was impossible because of the way Basil had to lay on the x-ray table. A test was possible using dye, but we all worried about a possible reaction to this dye. Both Basil's grandmas had experienced severe negative reactions to that kind of dye previously when they had undergone medical testing. I also had suffered a bad reaction. The doctor believed it was too risky, plus he knew there was nothing that could be done, anyway. Dr. Timmons said the best thing to do for Basil would be to get him back home in his own bed with familiar surroundings and nurses he knew because the time of life for Basil was running short.

As soon as Basil became stable enough to leave Ohio, we came home. Dr. Timmons was not mistaken about Bubby. He had no appetite, and would not eat. He tried a bite of food every now and then, but he never ate another meal. He had to have an IV solution for nourishment the rest of his life.

We all prepared for the worst. After hearing the latest report from Dr. Timmons, Priscilla considered coming home from Ohio. Bubby started asking for PJ, so she decided to come home immediately. Once she got home, she spent all of her time with us; she went nowhere. Even though she didn't want to believe that she would actually lose her brother, deep down I believe she knew it was inevitable. Basil, Sr. went about his daily work routine. Although he knew we were losing our son, he buried himself in his work so he would not have to face reality.

A MOTHER'S PERSPECTIVE

During this period, although I was frantically busy, I gave some thought to the life we'd all had together. Mothers everywhere have special memories of their children—some good, some funny, and some not-so-good. I'm no different. Most of our normal days were pretty much like other people's. Before Bubby got so sick, the hardest thing for me to do was to go grocery shopping. It was nearly impossible to take him along, because I couldn't put him in a cart like other children. Even something falling against him could hurt Basil or even break a bone. When I needed to go to the store, most of the people who could take care of Basil were at work or school. So I had to do my shopping when the others were available. Mom helped me out a lot by shopping for me. Our days were fairly routine—getting up, getting dressed, eating meals, bathing at night, and the special times of visiting with friends or playing games. When he didn't have school the next day, we would often stay up later to watch a movie or play Nintendo games. Then we both had the luxury of sleeping in the next day! The first thing we had to do each morning was wash his face and hands, dress him, and comb his hair. He was very particular about being clean and looking nice. One morning that sticks out in my mind, I had just dressed Bubby and was carrying him into his chair for breakfast. I hadn't taken the time to get dressed myself, so I was still wearing my long robe. In our house we had a step up into our family room, and as I stepped up, I tripped on my robe and fell with Bubby. It was awful; I tried to protect Basil, but he ended up breaking his leg. He was more worried about me than he was his leg. I was crying because I felt so bad; he patted my face with his little hand and said, "It's OK, honey, you only broke my leg." I know he intended to make me feel better, but he was so sweet about it that I think I cried even more.

Whenever he had broken limbs, bathing became very difficult. If he had a broken arm, I could usually manage the bath by myself. I would rest the injured arm on my arm and carry him into the bathroom. Sometimes he could even help hold the broken arm. But a broken leg was a different matter. It took two of us to carry him into the bathroom. I would have to fold a washcloth and put it under his leg to support it. After his bath, Priscilla or Basil Sr. would help me carry him back out. We just had to be extra careful until the broken bone had a chance to heal, which usually took ten to fourteen days.

As a mom, I have certain special family memories of our times with Bubby; some of them were funny and some were serious. One of the funniest times was a trick Bubby played on us. One day when he was about fourteen years old, I decided to take a nap on the couch. I put Basil on the floor beside me. When I woke up, Basil was gone! Now, remember, this was a child who could not walk or crawl. I was terrified. I called out, "Basil Jr., where are you?" At first I thought that somehow he had scooted over towards an open stairway we had leading into our basement. I called for Priscilla to see if she had taken him, but she hadn't. We looked everywhere in that huge family room. Then we heard a familiar little snicker. We followed the sound of that snicker and found him squeezed in between our patio door and the TV. The patio curtain hid him from view. He was so happy because he was finally able to hide from us all by himself! When we picked him up, he bit down on his little finger and laughed and laughed. He had to laugh that way to prevent the breaking of any ribs. This little episode earned him a new nickname; his dad found out about this later and decided to call him a "Scooter Frog" because he had scooted his tiny body all over that room. His daddy called him "Frog" many times after that!

Another time when Bubby was about a year old, Priscilla was trying to play with him. She was playing "house" and she wanted to include her little brother. She decided to hang a small purse on his arm; he held out his arm, she put on the purse, and his arm broke. Both of them were crying by the time I got there. Priscilla's heart was broken because she had hurt her baby brother. But she loved to spend time with Bubby. As they got older, they played together for hours. When she got home from school, she'd pick him up and off they'd go to her room to play. Basil often said he was helping her with her homework! They even did dishes together. Basil would sit on the counter while P.J. (short for Priscilla Jean) washed the dishes. She'd even give him something small and light to dry so he'd feel like he was helping, too. They had a real bond of closeness between them, maybe even closer than if they had both been healthy.

Sometimes things happened unexpectedly that could have ended with tragic results. This happened when Basil first got sick. He was taking morphine by mouth at that time. He wanted to hold the spoon and give it to himself, so I let him. Suddenly he began gasping for air. I grabbed him and ran towards the back door because Basil Sr. and Gary were working outside. Luckily, my niece, Leah, was there to open the door for me. I screamed for Basil to come. Somehow I got down on my knees with him, and with Basil's help, I managed to flip Bubby over so we could pat his back. It worked, and we were able to save him. I know that kids often choke, but this was especially dangerous because I could not have held him and opened the door by myself, he could have broken ribs, or we could have hurt him as we patted his back. While we were able to save him, I believe that things started changing for the worse after that. I've often wondered if he didn't aspirate on some of the morphine then. Scary moments like that are especially difficult with a child like Basil.

Sometimes I wonder what effect all of this has had on Priscilla. She had to watch her brother suffer so much, and I know she had to dwell on the thought of whether her brother would live or not. That's a heavy burden for a young girl to carry. She never resented her brother in any way, even though I always had to put Bubby's needs first. Priscilla was a tremendous help when she got older. She could then stay with Basil, bathe him, fix his meals, and do as much for him as I did. A lot of times Basil even wanted P.J. to do things for him instead of me. I'm sure many people wonder how we managed to find time for Priscilla. That never seemed to be a problem. None of us felt cheated in any way because of the amount of time Bubby required. Priscilla was in Brownies, dance lessons, and she had birthday parties like other kids. Basil went right along with us when we took her to meetings or lessons. We even encouraged her to play basketball her freshman year in high school when she showed an interest in the sport. We bought the shoes, took her to all of the practices, and cheered her on. But she decided it was more work than fun, and she really didn't want that kind of work! When P.J. got her license, she often took Bubby with her. The first time she did that without me along seemed like a long, long time even though I had told her to be back in an hour. I had such a "worry" headache—the kind mothers are used to. But it all went well, and Basil loved being with his sister. I guess I started to realize that even though Basil was in a tiny body, he had the mind and attitudes of a teenager. He enjoyed having bits of independence and time away from me. When Priscilla started dating, she and her date often took Bubby shopping and to card shops to trade baseball cards. They enjoyed spending time together; Basil missed her so much when she moved to Ohio after high school. She had a job there, and lived there about a year and a half. This was during the time Bubby was so sick, but P.J. called him often and came home for frequent visits.

One of my most memorable times was Mothers' Day in May of 1992. Basil secretly sent his dad to Fort Wayne to get me a special meal from one of our favorite restaurants. He was so thrilled to think that he had surprised me, even though he couldn't eat a bite himself. Just before this, he had received his first and only credit card. He was so proud to have a card in his name; he couldn't wait to buy me something. As soon as his Aunt Nora got here from Ohio, he sent her on a special mission. He had seen a ring in a jewelry store flier that he wanted to get me. He gave his credit card to Nora, and sent her to Fort Wayne to buy me a mother's ring. Nora found the ring and got it for him. The store wrapped it up so prettily for them. I was surprised and touched by his thoughtful gift. The ring is onyx with gold letters spelling "Mom." It has a tiny diamond chip in it, which I'm sure is what caught his eye. He loved those diamonds! He put it on my finger, kissed my finger, and said, "Mom, you're the best mom in the world." I treasure that moment.

During all the days of Basil's sickness, there were some unpleasant moments. I guess the main problem I faced during those times was the attitude that seemed to come from some members of the medical profession about kids with disabilities. The attitude seems to say that these kids may not need the best possible medical attention because they're probably not going to live long, anyway. I know it's hard to believe anyone could feel that way, but I found it to be true. We faced this situation with one doctor. This doctor didn't always see Basil, but he seemed to make quick, and sometimes bad, decisions when he did see Basil. Bubby had been having severe headaches which caused him to vomit. I called the doctor, and he said he'd order some medication to control the vomiting. When Nora returned home from the pharmacy, I saw that the medicine was one that Bubby was allergic to. Apparently the doctor had not even checked Basil's medical records. My nurse called the doctor, and explained that this medication could not be given to Basil because of his allergy. The doctor said he'd get something else ready, so Nora went back to town to get it. Since Nora had some experience working with patients on strong medications, she recognized this one as something that should not be given with large doses of morphine. We all got out our book on prescriptions and their side effects and interactions (PDR). It confirmed what Nora thought to be true. My nurse again called the doctor; he wasn't too happy to hear from us again. I guess he was upset because we were questioning his decision. He and my nurse had a verbal battle on the phone. I was sitting across the table from the nurse, and I could hear him tell her not to question his authority, but to give the medicine in the exact dosage that he prescribed. The nurse was a little scared to administer that drug, but we decided to dilute it before we gave it to Bubby. After we gave it to him, I tried to rest on the couch since Nora and the nurse were with Basil. Nora kept saying something was wrong. She didn't think Basil was acting like himself. I heard them talking, so I hurried into the other room to see what was wrong. Immediately, I knew something wasn't right. This time, I called Bubby's regular doctor (at home) and she said she would meet us at the hospital. Basil's tongue was swelling, he was turning blue around his nose and mouth, and he was shaking. The reaction even caused his back to arch. I remember Bubby saying how scared he was as his dad drove us to the hospital. I kept reassuring him that Dr. Fischer would be there, and everything was going to be OK. When we got to the hospital, she had to give him another drug to counter the effects of this one. We also had to admit him, so that was yet another hospital stay. I know that Basil Jr. would have died that night if Dr. Fischer hadn't met us at the hospital, or if we had not diluted that drug. It seemed whenever we had to deal with that other doctor, things never turned out well. I try to understand that doctors get overworked, and that it can't be pleasant getting calls in the middle of the night; however, when a child is suffering, that is not pleasant for the child or the parents. It appears that some medical professionals tend to take the situation too lightly when a disabled child is involved. The parents know the whole situation, and the seriousness of it. Maybe this type of professional just hasn't developed the compassion necessary to meet the needs of a disabled child and his family.

My advice to those medical professionals is to not accept the responsibility of treating disabled children if they cannot handle it. I guess to be fair I should mention that Dr. Fischer had personal reasons for being so understanding. She and her husband had four of their own children, plus they had adopted two kids with disabilities. She knew what it was like to have a sick child with nurses in the home. Maybe those parents with disabled children ought to look for a doctor with that kind of compassion. I do realize that Basil Jr. was hard to doctor. He was eighteen, and yet he had the body of an infant. That combination has to be difficult to treat. Even doctors who deal with disabilities all the time might have trouble treating a patient like Bubby. But when it's your child and you are in a battle to keep him alive and well, it becomes a tense situation. This is especially true for a mother like me who truly loved her child. I am a strong believer in God; I believe that He is the one who has control over our number of days on earth. But I also believe that doctors should work hard to give the best possible health care to any patient while God has given that patient life to live.

OUR TALK BEFORE DEATH

After our last visit to Nora's, Basil's appetite simply stopped. We went on this way for about six weeks. Life for my son changed very rapidly; his head pain was worse, his legs ached and jerked a lot, and his stomach quit functioning. Basil vomited and heaved often to the extent that he couldn't brush his teeth, or take a drink. Dr. Fischer asked Basil if he wanted a food supplement put through his central line. Basil knew the danger of the line getting clogged; he also knew that he would not get the morphine if that happened; and he knew that he could not stand the pain without the morphine. Instead of giving a negative answer, Basil simply changed the subject and asked Dr. Fischer if she had seen his new Simpson family figures. Dr. Fischer was very upset because she told me that Basil was literally starving to death; yet, she respected his wishes. All that could be done for him was to give him breathing treatments, change the ice packs on his head, put the heating pad on and off his legs as he asked, and do what we could to keep him comfortable. Priscilla even took some time off work so she could come home to be with Bubby.

Seeing my son go through all his suffering the last few weeks of his life made me realize that Melba, the nurse who had a heart-to-heart with me, was absolutely right.

Basil and I needed to have a heart-to-heart talk and say our goodbyes soon. I knew Basil well enough to know that if I was patient he would soon get on the subject of getting better and telling me not to worry about his headache and all the morphine he was getting. I will probably recall the conversation Basil Jr. and I had on Thursday evening, May 7, 1992, every day for the rest of my life. I can still hear him saying, "Mom, when I get better . . . "and I stopped him from finishing his sentence. Today I still wonder what he was going to say to me, but I knew deep in my heart that what I had to say to him was more important to us both than anyone could ever imagine.

What I said to my son that night was the hardest thing that I have done in my lifetime. I sat by the side of Basil's bed, holding his little hand with tears flowing down my cheeks. I told him God had given us eighteen wonderful years to be together and that now God was waiting for him in heaven with open arms. As I told him all his pain and suffering would be over in heaven and he'd have peace and joy forever with God, Basil looked at me with those big brown eyes, as tears trickled down his face and said, "Oh, Mommy, what will you do without me?" At that time I promised my precious son that it didn't matter how difficult things would be for me that I would go on with my life and try to be a good person in the eyes of God. Then some day we would be together again in Heaven where life with God would be perfect for us both. We hugged and kissed each other, holding on to one another for some time. As I wiped away his tears, we made our last promise to each other—as I would look up toward him every day, he'd be looking down at me. That night was the first and last time this conversation would be discussed. Our last days went on as usual. I knew when I told Basil Jr. that there was no hope of getting better, that I was thankful Priscilla had decided to come home from Ohio. Once his sister got home, nobody could do things for him quite like P.J.

On May 12th at 3:20 PM my son died. This was just a couple of days after our special Mothers' Day together. I had told Bubby not to be afraid when the time came because God was ready for him, and I would be there holding his hand until God reached for it. As death was so near, my son spoke in a loud voice. His last words were, "Take me home." At the time my son was passing away, a terrible storm came up. It sounded as if the roof was going to blow off, but as life left his tiny body, everything became quiet and still, almost supernaturally.

When I had realized how sick Basil was and that he didn't have much time here on earth, every night in my prayers I would ask God to please give me a sign when Bubby died that he was in Heaven. I'm sure the quietness during the storm was my sign that Basil was safe with God. My knowing that my son is not suffering, but happy in Heaven has helped me survive these long and empty days here on earth, and has made me much closer to God.

Dr. Fischer was notified when Basil became cyanotic and was having trouble breathing. She told me to raise his oxygen and give him a breathing treatment, which his nurse and I were doing. Priscilla ran next door to get our neighbor, Deb Johns, who works in respiratory therapy, to help us. Dr. Fischer came out to the house but my son survived only a few minutes after she arrived. As Basil took his last breath, my body became numb and weak, but I will never forget the ache I felt in my heart.

Basil and I had said our goodbyes, so I felt it necessary to leave the room for a few minutes so my husband and daughter could do the same in the silence of the room where my son lay.

After a few minutes, I went back into his room; while standing by his bed all I could think about was what a wonderful son he had been and all the terrific memories he had left with us. I knew the funeral director, Howard Rich, would soon be coming for him, so I moved him to a fresh spot on his bed, and then disconnected Basil from the machines, washed him, and put his favorite IU gown on him.

When Mr. Rich arrived, my husband and I sat down at the kitchen table with him and discussed the time of Bubby's viewing and funeral. The time came for Basil to be put on the stretcher; I asked Mr. Rich if it was all right for me to carry him to the dining room and lay him on it. Mr. Rich said that it was unusual, but if I wanted to, it was perfectly all right with him. I remember so vividly as I picked up my son's small, fragile body, thinking how precious he was and how everyone would miss his presence and laughter in our home. When I laid him down, I covered him with his favorite IU blanket. My husband and daughter kissed him goodbye, as I did, before he was taken away from his home for the final time.

The next few days, everything seemed unreal to me; the day of Basil's funeral is a clear memory, though. As we took him past our house for the last time and down State Road 218 to the cemetery, I'll always remember the farmers in the fields stopping their tractors, taking off their hats, and bowing their heads as if praying when we drove by. It made the tears run down my face as I thought what wonderful people we have around us. They touched my heart in a way I'll always remember the rest of my life.

Priscilla stayed with us another week or so after Bubby's funeral. Then she went back to Ohio and her job, eventually, however, returning home to live. I really believe P.J. has a big empty spot in her life since her brother died. As her mother, it seems to me that she can't find real contentment in her life. I guess we all deal with grief differently. I'm so thankful for the close relationship she and Basil Jr. had; I know Basil would want P.J. to be happy.

Only seventeen days after Basil's death, the senior class of Bluffton High School, Basil's class of 1992, was graduating. Even though Basil had to graduate early due to his severe pain, he was not forgotten when it came to his class of '92. Graduation was dedicated to the memory of Basil W. Rhodes, Jr., on the 29th day of May, 1992. Although it was difficult, Basil Sr. and I attended the graduation ceremony. Mike and Deb Johns, as well as Deb Johnson, sat with us. I knew Bubby would have wanted us there; he would have loved the dedication the class made. There is now a "Friends of Basil Rhodes, Jr." scholarship fund at our local bank. This was started in May 1992 by Joe and Mike Smekens. Each May this scholarship is awarded to a college-bound graduating senior from Bluffton High School through the local unit of Dollars for Scholars. I'm sure the students who receive this scholarship will be very appreciative for the help to further their education; and who knows—maybe if they end up at IU, they will give an extra cheer in memory of one of the biggest fans of them all.

BRAVE FINAL DAYS

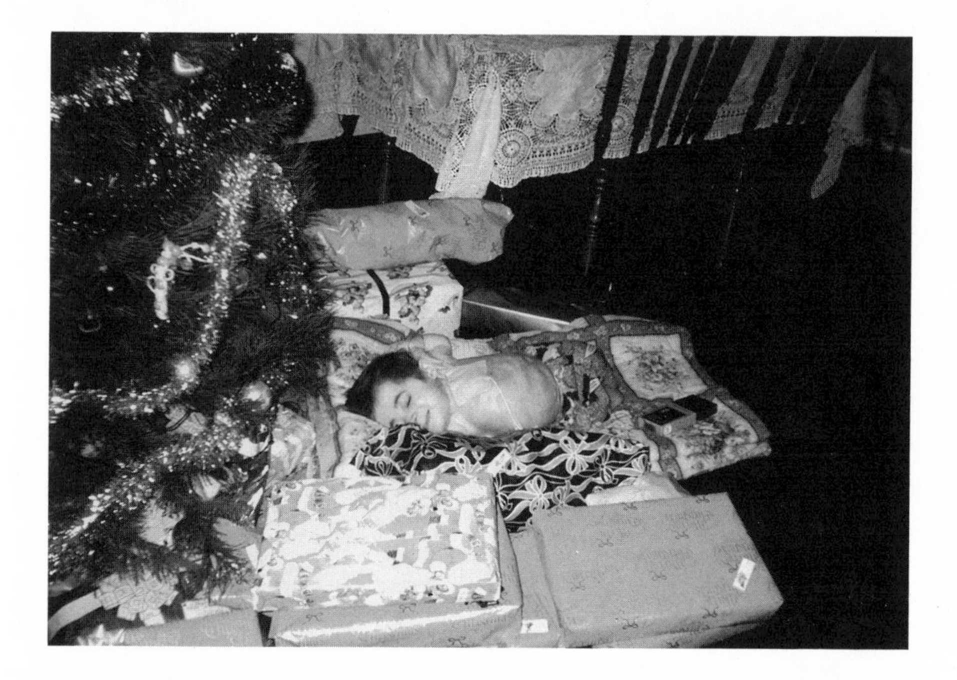

On Christmas December 25, 1991, his last, Basil looks weary.

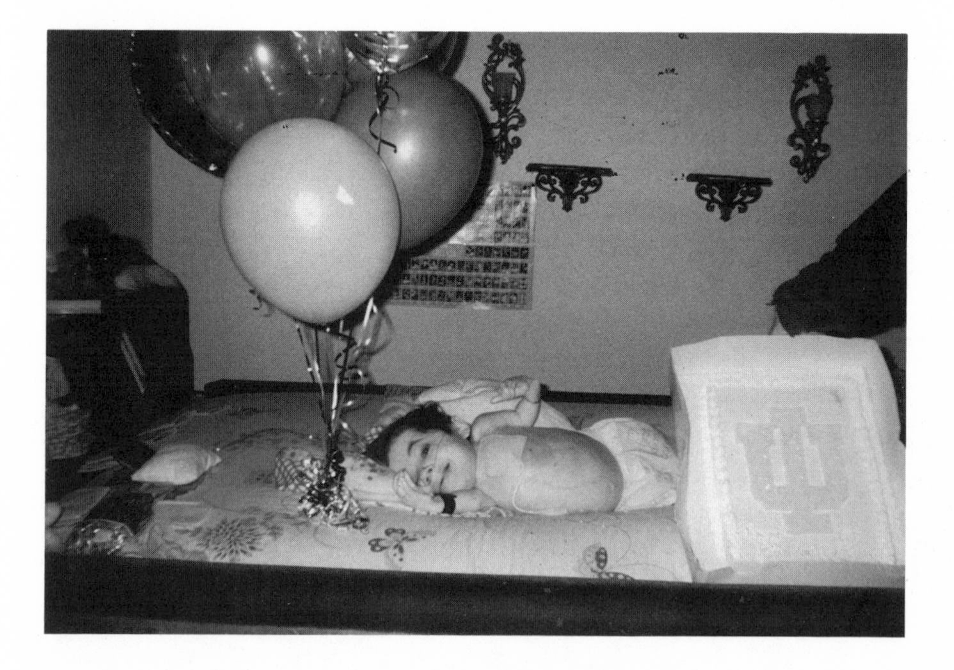

March 4, 1992 marked Basil's birthday with IU symbols.

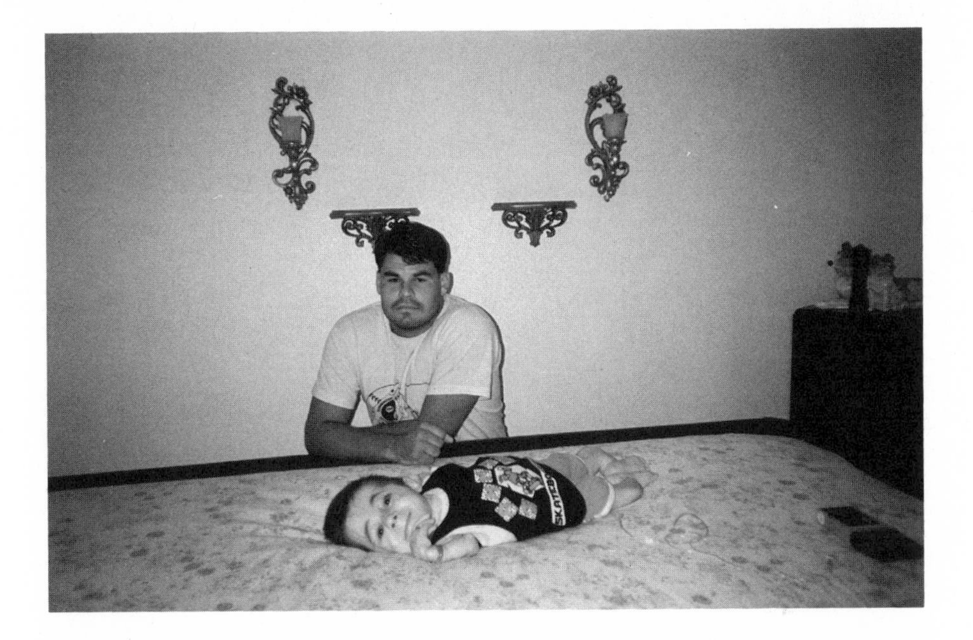

Tom Brickley was the person responsible for putting Basil's name in for the Young Heroes' Medal of Honor Award.

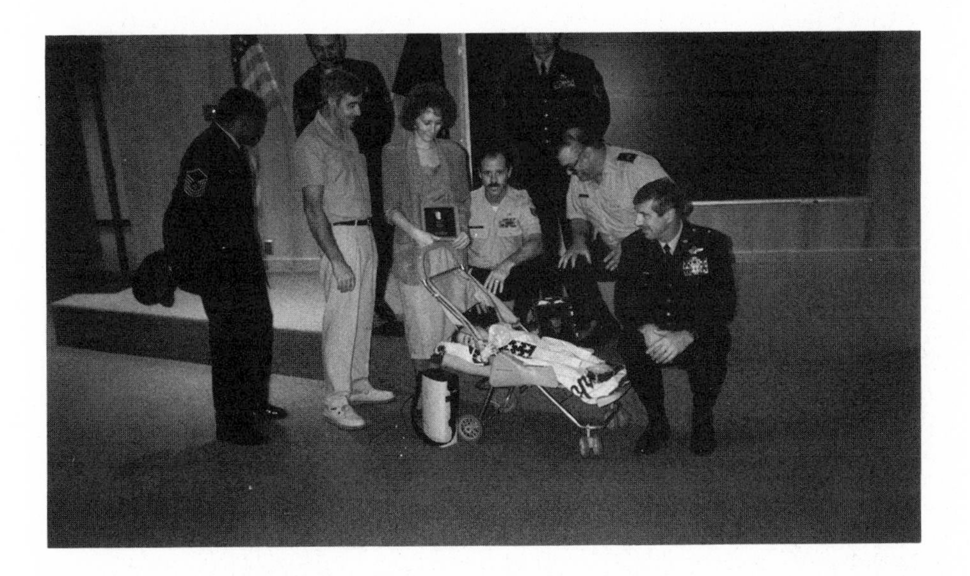

On August 28, 1991 at Fort Wayne, Indiana Air Base, Basil received his Young Heroes' Medal of Honor Award.

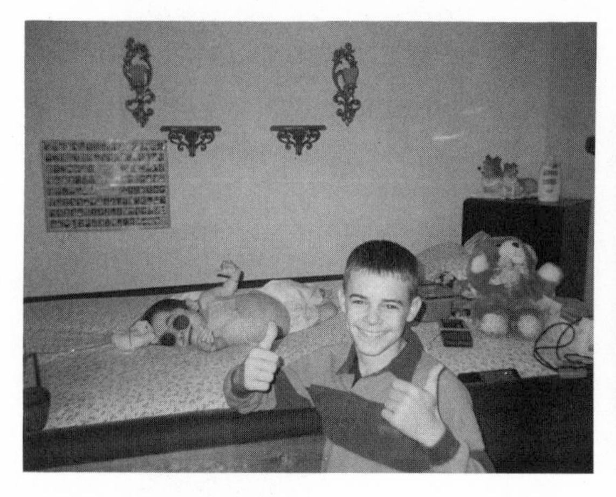

Brady Johns was a neighbor and good friend.

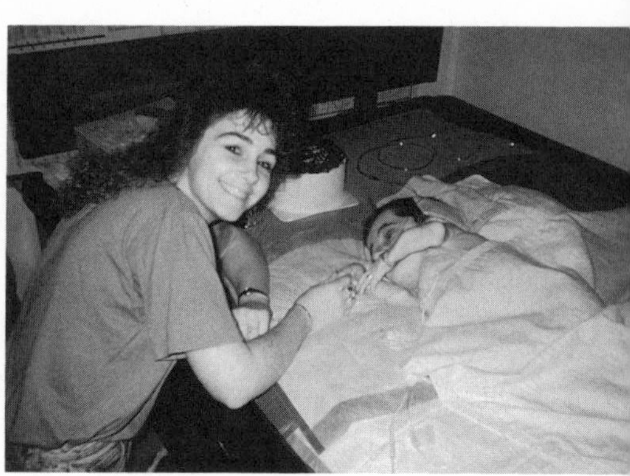

Basil is shown presenting his sister the bracelet he bought for her 21st birthday.

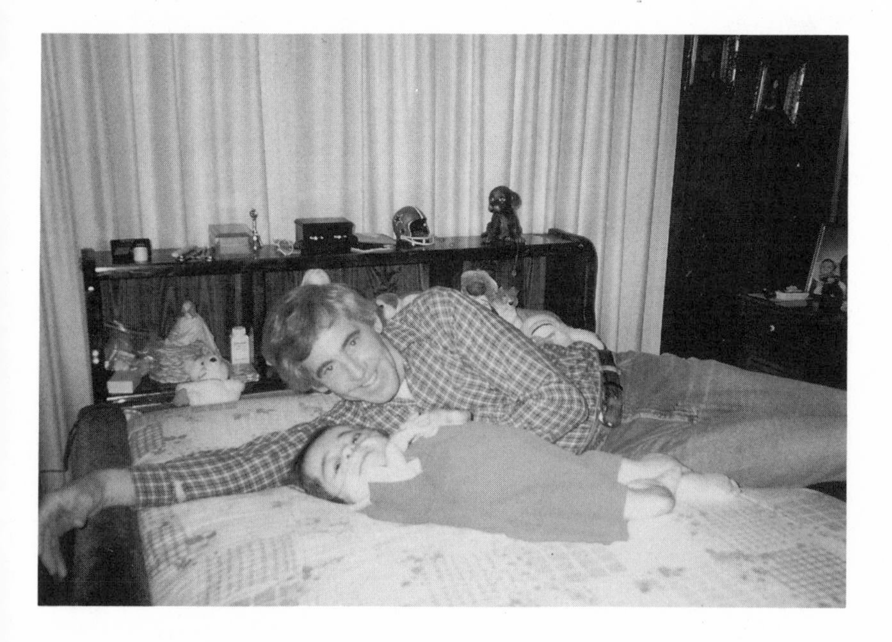

Basil and his Dad both had a smile for the camera.

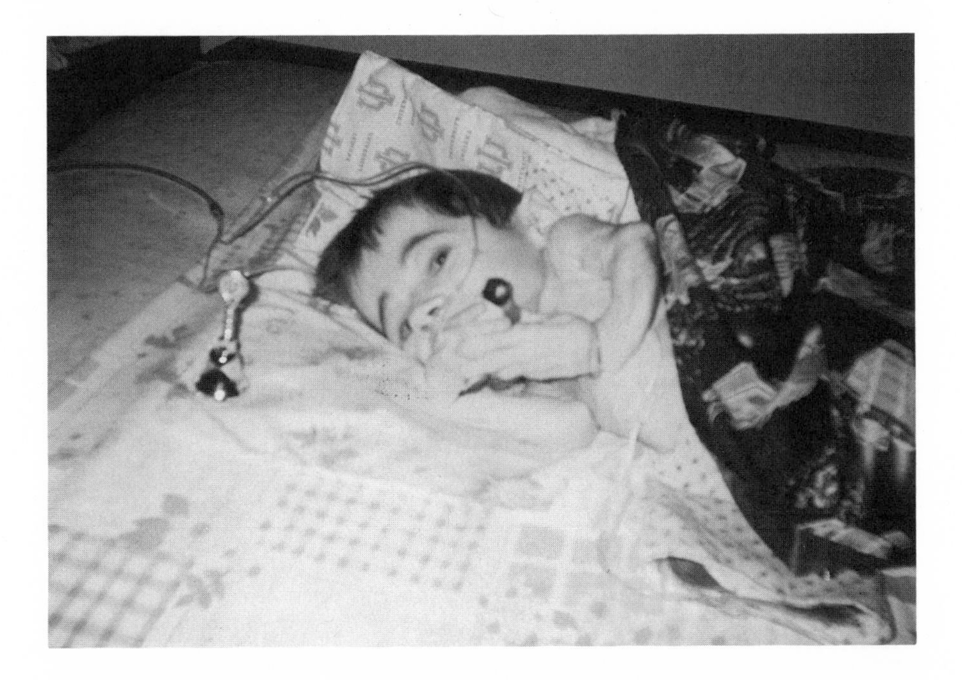

Basil's bird Sunshine had some of the physical freedom his master missed.

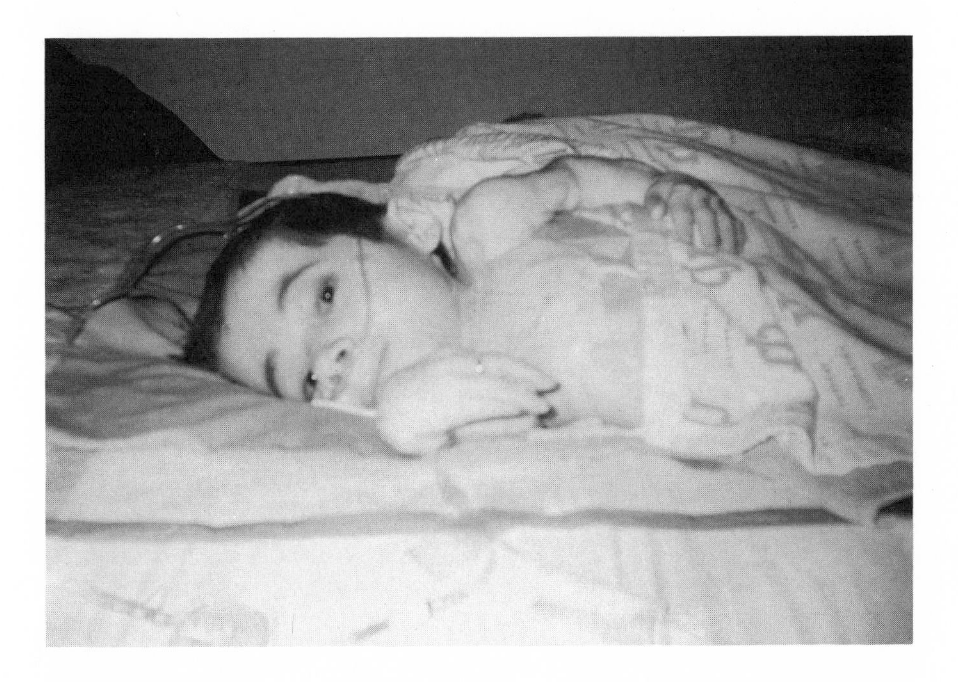

Basil, shown just seven days before his death on May 12, 1992.

EPILOGUE

Since I had promised Bubby that I would go on with my life, I knew I had to keep that promise. I waited about a year and a half before making any decisions. First of all, I had to allow time for grieving. Any parent who loses a child has a difficult time adjusting. Basil and I had such a special relationship because we were together most of the time; actually, my life revolved around my son. When he was gone, my life seemed empty and without a purpose. As time went on, though, I remembered my promise. One day I thought I was cleaning house, but I was actually tearing things up more than cleaning. My neighbor, Ellen, stopped in and said, "Dorothy, whatever are you doing?"

I realized then that I really didn't know what I was doing.

And I knew it was time to find some purpose in my life again. I had been going to the graveyard every day to visit his grave. I felt I had to do that, yet I knew it was just a constant reminder of my loss. I was really close to depression, and I had developed some health problems, too.

I knew I wanted to do something I liked, was good at, and that I could do on my own. I had always enjoyed "playing" with hair, and I was pretty good at it. I thought if I had my own shop, I would be my own boss and not have the stress of working for someone else. So I decided to go to barber school in Ohio. Since I doctored in Ohio, I often stayed with Nora when I had to see my doctor. In October of 1993, I started classes. I stayed with Nora; I would come home some weekends, and Basil would come to Ohio the other weekends. That was quite a stressful time! When I did get home, there were bills to be paid, laundry to do, and many people to see. It was pretty hectic. I developed a way of studying during those long drives to and from Ohio. I wrote questions out, folded the paper, and had the answers on the other side. It may not have been the best thing to do while driving, but it helped me with my classes.

It took me a year to complete barber school. We already had a building in Bluffton that Basil was remodeling for my shop. I knew I had to be in town in order to be available to the customers and make barbering pay. By the time I finished school, Basil was just finishing the inside of the shop. Then began the long process of my getting my Indiana license, a shop license, and a license to sell the products I had chosen to sell. It seemed like it took too long to get all of that, but I was finally able to open "DJ's Barber Shop" in March of 1995. I was so nervous about opening up and not having enough customers. I only had to worry about that for a short time; after the first month, I seem to have a pretty full schedule!

It really helped me out to be able to stay with John and Nora. I met a lot of new friends in Ohio, and it sure made me focus on something else. I enjoy my work, and I know that while I'll never get over missing Basil Jr., at least I've kept my promise to him.

Deb Johnson ended up getting a full time teaching position at Bluffton High School, teaching English and reading. She believes her relationship teaching Basil helped the corporation get to know her. She still talks to her students about Basil.

I want to personally thank all the wonderful people of Bluffton and Wells County. Their support and encouragement have been truly appreciated. The community was so kind in setting up a fund to buy Basil Jr. a computer. It was that computer that he used for school and his own personal enjoyment. I especially want to thank Jim Brown for assisting us in the preparation of the disc of the manuscript. I also want to thank the doctors and nurses at the Caylor-Nickel Clinic for their excellent and personal care of Basil. I appreciate Nancy New for being Basil's personal barber for eighteen years; I value her friendship, too. I want to thank all of our friends and neighbors for their continued support. I know they'll always remember Basil and the lift he gave all our lives. And every day as I look up, I know my angel is looking down at me—and his wings are no longer broken.

Appendix

Basil Sr.'s parents are Leon and Violet Rhodes. They had eight children, but Oren passed away in 1962 from accidental carbon monoxide poisoning. The surviving children are Elsie, Wanda, Jack, Basil, Gary, Arles, and Judy. All of them still live in West Virginia, except Wanda who lives in Clearwater, Florida, and Gary who lives in Bluffton, Indiana, just a few miles from where we live. My parents are Sarah Harmon and Everett Raines. My dad still lives in West Virginia and is remarried to Sherlyn. They have one child together, my half-sister, Donna Sue. A few years after their divorce, my mother married Frank Harmon, but they had no children. I have four brothers and sisters—Nora, Jim, Ann, and Donnie. Nora and Jim both live in Akron, Ohio, where my mother now resides. Frank passed away in 1986; since Mom's health is failing, she now lives with Nora. Ann still lives in West Virginia in the same house we bought from Leon. Donnie lives in southern Ohio.

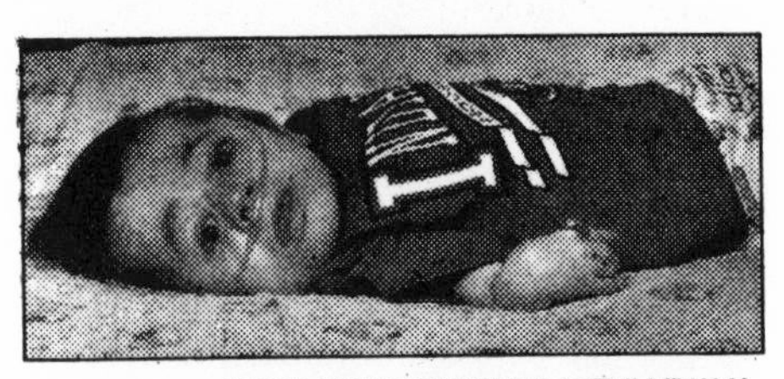

STAFF PHOTOGRAPH BY AKEMI MIYAMA

17-year-old sports fan Basil Rhodes.

Disorder can't slow sports fan

ROCKFORD, REIFFSBURG — The minute hand has edged past 12, and now it is heeling over, slowly and slowly, toward 7:05 in the evening. It is almost showtime here at Basil Rhodes' house.

"OK, Basil, we've got about three minutes until the show starts," says Art Saltsberg, gently, to the tiny figure on the bed. "We'll be calling on you for comments on a lot of subjects. We billed you as our tri-host tonight, Basil."

"I won't make you look bad or anything," Basil replies in his high, small child's voice.

No. He will not. He knows his sports forward, backward and sideways, especially if you want to talk about the Mets. He knows WOWO SportsTalk. He has called it so often that his co-hosts

BEN SMITH

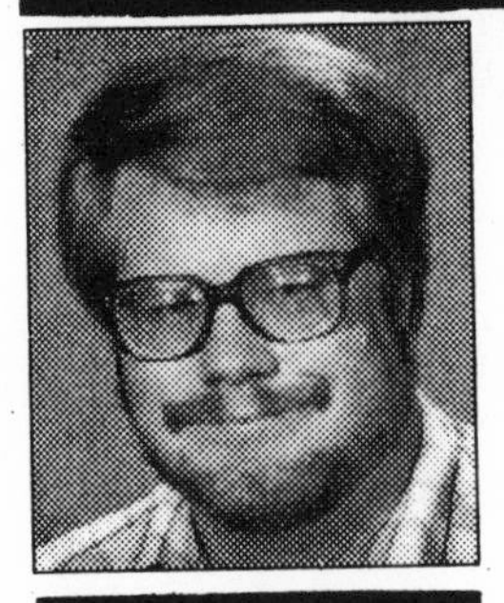

aren't Mr. Saltsberg and Mr. Pantazi to him. They're just plain Art and Dean.

"He thinks the world of those two guys," says his mom, Dorothy. "It's 'Art and Dean, Art and Dean,' you know."

So he is ready. A microphone has been pushed close to his head. The wires snake across the floor, joined by a number of clear plastic tubes. They are the tubes that connect Basil Rhodes, who is 17 years old and the size of an infant, to the big stainless steel oxygen tank that sits around the corner from his room.

"I wasn't sure how well this would go, because he was really sick earlier in the day," Dorothy is saying. "But I gave him a little extra medicine, and he's feeling pretty good now."

He is ready.

Osteogentsis imperfecta is not going to stop this, just as it didn't stop Basil Rhodes from becoming a high school graduate, just as it doesn't keep the sunny side out of his disposition.

Osteogentsis imperfecta is the medical term for Rhodes' condition, a ten-dollar word for being imprisoned by one's own body. It is a rare ailment in which the the bones never harden and grow, leaving the patient bedfast and endlessly susceptible to injury. Simply rolling over wrong can break ribs.

Basil has had osteogentsis imperfecta since birth. He suffers blinding headaches, and is in nearly constant pain that requires copious amounts of medication to control. The only escape is Nintendo, when he's feeling well enough, and sports. Lots of sports.

"He watches a lot of sports," Dorothy says. "The TV is always on when there's sports on. But he's at the point now where he can't really watch TV or anything because of the pain."

Yet he perseveres.

The doctors said he would only live three weeks, but he has lived and survived and even conquered, in a sense. With the aid of tutors, he graduated ninth in his Bluffton High School class this year. He won an award in 10th grade for getting the highest score on a standardized government test.

But sports remain his first love, and so this is his big night. With the help of Make A Wish Foundation of Northeast Indiana, Saltsberg and Pantazi and WOWO have come to Basil's house in Reiffsburg, a few miles south of Bluffton, to do SportsTalk.

Art and Dean, coming to him. This is big.

Right away, he is all over Pantazi about his Mets polishing off Dean's Cubs. He wonders if Dwight Gooden, Basil's main man, had a hand in it.

"No, Gooden didn't pitch in this series," Pantazi says.

"They didn't even need Gooden," Basil replies.

Pantazi reacts with mock indignation.

"Listen to this, he's starting already!" he cries. "This is going to be hard to take."

Art and Dean and Basil. They chat like best buddies, as airtime draws near. Dean chides Basil about the Mets and their Hands of Stone fielders. Basil agrees they "need four outfielders." The talk, easy and pleasant, flows on.

Suddenly it is time.

"Good evening," Saltsberg says smoothly. "Art and Dean with you tonight talking sports of all sorts until 8 o'clock. We're at a special location tonight. We're about six miles south of Bluffton in our good buddy Basil Rhodes' living room. Basil's going to be our co-host as we take you up until 8 o'clock talking about everything — including that Cubs' loss to the Mets today."

Basil crows. Dean cringes.

"Oh, you're gonna start already, right?" he says, and the show is on.

They cover the gamut in the next hour, Art and Dean and Basil. Mets-Cubs. The Komets' playoff payoff. Auto racing coverage. The NBA playoffs.

Basil talks as well as he can, having the time of his life. He thinks the Lakers will beat Portland. He doesn't think either his Mets or Saltsberg's Reds will win their respective divisions. He thinks Bob Knight, whom he once met, is a pretty OK guy.

"I think he's nice," Basil says. "I just don't think people see that side of him."

"Did he offer you a scholarship?" Dean asks.

"No, I was only in eighth or ninth grade when I met him," Basil answers. "Maybe he'll offer me one now."

That will never happen, of course. Osteogentsis imperfecta has seen to that. But it has also seen to a few other things.

You listen to Basil talk about his heroes, all those marvelous athletes, and you think maybe the adulation is going the wrong way. Maybe they should be talking about Basil: Basil who was only supposed to live three weeks; Basil who has a high school diploma and an outlook on life that is frankly remarkable under the circumstances.

"He's a very happy young man," Dorothy says. "Very, very seldom does he get upset. If there's something he wants to do really badly, and he's got one of his severe headaches, he gets a little flustered. Just like all of us would, I suppose."

There is nothing flustered about him now, though. The minute hand is edging toward 12, slowly and slowly, and it is almost 8 o'clock in the evening. Art and Dean and Basil are wrapping up.

"Thank you," Basil says quietly.

"Thank you, too," Pantazi answers.

And then, softly from the bed: "Can I do the closing?"

Sure. The closing to Basil's story is in the other room, where portraits of him abound, the largest of which hangs over the TV set. And if you shift your eyes a few inches, to the top of the television, you will find a small stack of VCR tapes there.

The one on top is "Rocky IV."

Life imitates art. Life, as Basil Rhodes must live it, is more compelling, more stirring, than art ever could be. There's your closing.

"This is WOWO," Basil says, as the minute hand hits 12. "For Art and Dean, this is Basil. Good night."

Ben Smith is a staff writer for The Journal-Gazette. His column appears Sunday, Tuesday, Thursday and Friday.

Putting Together the Puzzle of Basil

(Editor's note: The following article on Basil Rhodes, who died Tuesday, was written by Bluffton High School junior Katie Inskeep for publication in the senior edition of the school newspaper, *The Comet*. Miss Inskeep is co-editor of the newspaper and also serves on the *Retrospect* yearbook staff. She is the daughter of Kent and Lana Inskeep).

By KATIE INSKEEP

Appearance, especially in the case of Basil Rhodes, can be deceiving. To look at Basil, one might think him weak. A teenage boy imprisoned in a toddler's body; a skeleton so fragile that rolling over may break bones; a disease - osteotengentis imperfecta - so fatal, that at 17, he far outlived his life expectancy of 3 weeks. That fact by itself eliminates the possibility of weakness. But what kept Basil going? The question demands a complex answer. It remains a puzzle that needs to be fitted together for our sake.

Maestro's Teacher

When Deb Johnson came to teach Basil in October of 1988, there were uncertain feelings on both sides. Having had a frustrating time with a previous teacher, Basil was down on himself. He needed a teacher who could look past his physical limitations and highlight his sharp, witty mind. The connection of Basil and Deb Johnson was made through the medium of Dr. Evelyn Priddy.

Working for 13 years as a teacher at East Side Elementary and five years as the Reading Coordinator, Priddy taught Basil math and computer literacy. In the fall of 1988, Johnson volunteered to help with kindergarten roundup and she met Dr. Priddy. Sometimes afterward, Priddy went to rent an apartment owned by - who else? - the Johnson's. Eventually, Priddy learned of Johnson's teaching degree and about her positive attitude through Johnson's husband.

Excuse the cliche - it was a match made in heaven.

Basil - always looking for humor.

Deb Johnson - always ready to give it out.

They flattered each other.

Johnson had been out of the classroom for a while, privately tutoring students. She was nervous. "He deserved something good. So, with fear and trepidation..." joked Johnson, she began teaching Basil. During the first week, Johnson began calling Basil "Maestro" - explaining that it was a term at one time exclusively musical, meaning genius. The term had gained a wider meaning - one that suited Basil perfectly. "I wanted him to feel good about himself," remarked Johnson.

Because of all the preparation required, teaching Basil drained her energy. Almost all of their classwork had to be done within their five hours a day as he was plagued by intense headaches, which made reading difficult for him. Yet he "put up with the pain to communicate," explained Johnson.

Broken bones were common to Basil. The family cat laid on his arm once and broke it. His disease prevented his bones from hardening, and he was very vulnerable to breaks. Putting casts on broken bones was an impossibility because their weight would only break more bones.

But there were bones that were scared: his jaw bones. Dr. Priddy had been teaching Basil when he put his hand to his face and said, "I just broke my jaw. The only thing I can do is talk and I just broke my jaw."

Basil was physically dependant on his family for nearly everything. As a result, his mental independence was vital. During his third year of high school, his health deteriorated and his pain increased. He had built up a tolerance to morphine - the only pain killer that helped. He had to take his medicine orally, which upset his stomach. Basil faced an enormous decision.

Whether or not to quit school.

Th day Basil talked to Mrs. Johnson about quitting is what she refers to as the "sad day". "We sat and talked and cried a lot. Basil said, "But two years, I can't cope with two years."

"I told him that if I thought it would stop the pain, I'd tell him to quit that minute. But it wouldn't," Johnson said.

When Mrs. Johnson left that evening, she didn't know if she would still have a job. But when she walked in the next morning, she saw him smiling, and knew that, for the time being, all was healed.

Teaching Basil was both difficult and rewarding. Health class proposed a special challenge: physical fitness. "How do you make that appropriate for a child who has never walked on his own two feet?" asked Johnson. So Johnson geared up in gym shoes and a sweatsuit in an effort to give Basil a better understanding of physical fitness. She demonstrated sit-ups and push-ups on the floor, but from his perch on the bed, he couldn't see the demonstration very well.

The memory of the chapter brings laughter to the two when they talk of it on videotape. Dr. Priddy, now a professor at Huntington College, recorded them in September of 1990 for one of her classes. Even on the dim tape, Basil shines. It is sometimes difficult to understand Basil's high-pitched, slightly slurred speech. Like most of his organs, his tongue is too big for his body. But Johnson interprets his witty comments in a way that is so casual, so smooth, that it seems like part of the conversation. "We could read each other perfectly," she said.

His actions on the tape offer a glimpse of his true self: lacing his fingers and cracking his knuckles as the interview gets underway, crowing with laughter at a hilarious memory-so much that his whole body would quiver. "Sometimes I was afraid he'd choke," admitted Johnson.

"His strength of character draws people to him," said Priddy. Nearly two years later, students who viewed the tape still inquire about him.

Steam of Consciousness

Basil's education was different from most high school students. As Priddy put it, his education was the "integration of the thought process." School wasn't math, then English, then history, then computer. It was each subject laced with a healthy dose of all others, connected by questions from Basil's inquisitive mind. "Basil didn't see those walls," said Priddy.

Priddy admitted that when she first began teaching Basil, she viewed him as about a seventh grader instead of a freshman. "He was patient with me," she said. Soon she learned that not only was he as smart as any freshman, he had a sense of humor she hadn't seen in many high school students. "Basil had a sheer appreciation of humor. He made me feel like a comedian," said Priddy.

Basil had a way with people. He sincerely cared what was going on in their lives. Chris Mettler met Basil their sophomore year. He was the captain of his homeroom candy sales in which Basil was the top seller. As a matter of fact, he was the top seller of the entire sophomore class.

An important friendship sprouted. "I didn't treat him any different," said Chris, "You don't core a relationship by pitying."

For nine years, Jeremy Johns has been friends with Basil. Ever since Priscilla, Jeremy's next door neighbor and Basil's older sister, brought Jeremy to meet him. Their conversations flowed over with sports - baseball cards and the Hoosiers. Basil was an avid fan of the Hoosiers. (He had met Bobby Knight.) Basil and Jeremy even skipped school once to go shopping at the mall for tapes. "We spent all his money in about forty-five minutes," Jeremy said.

Many people credit Basil's family for his extraordinary life. "I never, ever heard her [Dorothy — Basil's mother] complain," said Johnson. Priddy called her a "saint".

"Mrs. Rhodes is the strongest person next to Basil I know," Chris related. "To handle that kind of adversary every forty-five seconds of a lifetime..." shaking his head slightly, he leaves the sentence without an ending.

Facing Realty

Graduation came quick for Basil. A whole year early, with one day's notice. He had been very ill, and was not expected to live through the night. Supt. McMillen was contacted. Within a matter of hours, Basil graduated ninth in his class, with an array of teachers, faculty, board members, and friends at his home to witness the ceremony. That night, Basil went into the hospital. He won again.

Johnson, though happy he graduated, was distraught. "It just stopped. I was a mess. I couldn't do anything." Finally, Priddy explained to her that she was in mourning. Mrs. Johnson was the only one who had lost Basil as a result of his graduation. "It took me three or four weeks of weaning away to get myself to where I could function," Johnson confessed.

Since Basil's birth, death had always lurked in the shadows. He had fought it, out-smarted it, for eighteen years. Love of his family and friends has been a great weapon, as had been his faith in God. God has always been a source of cohesion between he and Johnson.

On a Saturday afternoon, near the time when ten days later, Basil would die at his home in Reiffsburg, Deb Johnson and Evelyn Priddy looked across the table at Traditions; they decided to tell me Basil's dream.

Basil had dreamed that he died and went to heaven. "But it's okay," he told his mother, "because you were there to tell Jesus how to hold me."